Automotive Scrap Recycling

Automotive Scrap Recycling: Processes, Prices, and Prospects

JAMES W. SAWYER, JR.

PUBLISHED BY RESOURCES FOR THE FUTURE, INC.
DISTRIBUTED BY THE JOHNS HOPKINS UNIVERSITY PRESS
BALTIMORE AND LONDON

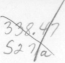

RESOURCES FOR THE FUTURE, INC.
1755 Massachusetts Avenue, N.W., Washington, D.C. 20036

Resources for the Future is a nonprofit corporation for research and education in the development, conservation, and use of natural resources and the improvement of the quality of the environment. It was established in 1952 with the cooperation of the Ford Foundation. Part of the work of Resources for the Future is carried out by its resident staff; part is supported by grants to universities and other nonprofit organizations. Unless otherwise stated, interpretations and conclusions in RFF publications are those of the authors; the organization takes responsibility for the selection of significant subjects for study, the competence of the researchers, and their freedom of inquiry.

This book is one of RFF's industry studies which are conducted under the quality of the environment program and directed by Allen V. Kneese and Blair T. Bower. It was edited by Ruth B. Haas. Charts were drawn by Clare and Frank Ford.

RFF editors: Mark Reinsberg, Joan Tron, Ruth B. Haas, Margaret Ingram

Copyright © 1974 by Resources for the Future, Inc.
All rights reserved
Manufactured in the United States of America

The Johns Hopkins University Press, Baltimore, Maryland 21218
The Johns Hopkins University Press Ltd., London

Library of Congress Catalog Card Number 74-3101
ISBN 0-8018-1620-3

Library of Congress Cataloging in Publication data
will be found on the last printed page of this book.

Contents

34455

Tables

Figures

ix

Preface

Interest in recycling has mushroomed in recent years, in response first to "environmental" concern and second to "resource exhaustion" concern. The closed-cycle economy has been put forth as the answer to both problems. However, to date there has been little rigorous analysis of the implications of different degrees of reuse of materials.

An analysis of recycling is a logical part of Resources for the Future's focus on residuals management in industry. Residuals represent a potential source of raw materials, an alternative to so-called "virgin materials." Nevertheless, the acquisition and processing of residuals to produce useful raw materials, be those residuals used newspapers or abandoned automobiles, involves energy and other material inputs and results in the generation of residuals, just as does the use of virgin materials.

Very often the analysis of the potential of residuals as raw materials has been in a physical–technological context, rather than in an economic one, that is, addressing explicitly economic supply and demand functions. The calculation of the supply of an available material, such as ferrous material, in residuals such as municipal mixed solid wastes, and the "evaluation" of that supply in terms of the unit, market price of ferrous material, after it has been processed, completely ignores the problems of original acquisition or collection of the residual, the costs of processing the residual, and the transportation of the output raw material to the places of use.

Sawyer includes all of these aspects in his analysis of one important type of residual, obsolete automobiles. Although the ferrous material derived from obsolete automobiles comprises a small proportion—3 or 4 percent—of total metallics feed to steel production in the United States, this type of residual is particularly important in terms of its "visibility"—impact on the visual quality of the environment. It is also important in terms of the social costs imposed by adandoned vehicles in major metropolitan areas.

Analysis of the disposition of obsolete automobiles is important in a more fundamental sense, in that this type of residual demonstrates the entire range of factors which determine the extent of reuse of a material over time—changing specifications on product outputs of steel; changing design of final products using steel, such as automobiles; technology of steel production; technology of residuals processing; and technology of residuals transportation. The technologic, economic, and socio-psychological aspects of final product characteristics are interwoven; the interaction is clearly shown in Sawyer's analysis.

The study represents the imaginative combination of formal mathematical models with primary data collection. The result of the analysis is to shed significant light on the elasticity of supply of ferrous scrap from obsolete automobiles and the implicit or explicit constraints on the demand for ferrous scrap. It provides a basis for evaluating the effects of various proposed governmental policies.

Blair T. Bower
Resources for the Future

December 1973

Acknowledgments

Professor Iraj Zandi originally suggested to me the possibility of applying a form of input–output technique to throw light on the steel scrap industry. I am grateful for the supervision he provided while I was preparing the doctoral dissertation that forms the nucleus of this work. I am also grateful to Resources for the Future, not only for funding the dissertation, but for the interest and enthusiasm I have received both as a Fellow and as a Research Associate. Blair Bower, Clifford Russell, and Jeff Vaughan in particular have cheerfully devoted substantial amounts of their time to reviewing this manuscript and working out problems of analysis. I am grateful for their comments and assistance as well as for the suggestions offered by Fred Wells.

In addition, I would like to thank the Institute of Scrap Iron and Steel (ISIS) for its assistance and the cooperation of many of its members whom I interviewed. They were more than generous with their time and confidential information. Special thanks go to J. Hayden Boyd of the Motor Vehicle Manufacturers Association, Calvin Lieberman of the ISIS, Harold J. Polta of the U.S. Bureau of Mines, and Frank Smith of the Environmental Protection Agency, all of whom devoted considerable time to careful review of the first draft of this manuscript.

My wife has patiently helped me with everything from computer programming to final proofreading. Without her interest it is doubtful that I would have completed the task. My editor, Ruth Haas, has been a great help in the arduous task of preparing this manuscript for publication and I am grateful for her efforts. Finally, I would like to thank Dee Stell of RFF for her rapid and accurate typing of the manuscript, and perhaps more importantly, for her patience with its many revisions.

J. W. Sawyer

December 1973

xiii

Introduction

Resources for the Future has for some time been studying the problem of residuals management.[1] In the initial studies, such as those of Spofford[2] and Russell,[3] the major objective was to develop a conceptual/analytic formulation of the problem, its significance to society, and its relation to other problems of concern to both industrial firms and society. Given this framework, RFF began studying various major industries to gain insight into residuals production by them and, more importantly, into the cost of residuals management in a given industry, that is, the cost of reducing residuals discharged into the environment. Studies have already been made on the beet sugar[4] and petroleum refining[5] industries. Other industries currently being studied include pulp paper and steel,[6] in addition to the work reported here on steel scrap.

---

[1] Residuals as an economic term can be defined in the following way. All economic activities consist of inflows and outflows of materials and energy. Some of the outflow will comprise the products that are the desired result of that activity. The rest of the outflows are residuals because they have zero prices in existing markets. A residual is thus a nonproduct output with zero price in the current market.

[2] W. O. Spofford, Jr., "Solid Residuals Management, Some Economic Considerations," *Natural Resources Journal*, vol. 11, pp. 561–589 (1971).

[3] C. S. Russell, "Models for Investigation of Industrial Responses to Residuals Management Actions," *Swedish Journal of Economics*, vol. 73, no. 1 (March 1971), pp. 134–156.

[4] George O. G. Löf and Allen V. Kneese, *The Economics of Water Utilization in the Beet Sugar Industry* (The Johns Hopkins Press for Resources for the Future, 1968).

[5] Clifford S. Russell, *Residuals Management in Industry* (The Johns Hopkins University Press for Resources for the Future, 1973).

[6] William J. Vaughan, "A Linear Programming Approach to Residuals Management in the Iron and Steel Industry," Ph.D. dissertation to be submitted to the Department of Economics, Georgetown University, 1974; see also Clifford S. Russell and W. J. Vaughan, "A Linear Programming Model of Residuals Management for Integrated Iron and Steel Production," to be published in the *Journal of Environmental Economics and Management*, vol. 1, no. 1.

It is intended that the results of the steel and the steel scrap industry studies will be combined at a future date to address the broad question of ferrous recycling discussed in this work.

The steel scrap industry has received very little detailed examination by either engineers or economists. The lack of background information made it necessary, in this study, to develop a qualitative description of the steel scrap industry and its methods of operation. A quantitative description of a major segment of the industry, namely, that associated with the conversion of obsolete automobiles into steel scrap, was then made and was formulated as two mixed integer linear programming problems.

The structure of the scrap processing industry is given in chapter 2; chapter 3 discusses the various ferrous scrap grades and the steel scrap quality problem. After this necessary background information, the remainder of the study follows the order of events in which a no longer useful automobile is transformed into processed scrap. Chapter 4 discusses the rate of automobile deregistration. A programming model of automobile dismantling is presented in chapter 5.

In chapter 6, following a discussion of the investment and operating costs of equipment used in processing dismantled automobiles into finished scrap, a programming model is presented of the steel scrap processing industry for a geographic region. This model uses as input data some of the information developed from the dismantling model. The two mathematical models are designed to cast light on such problems as the supply of steel scrap made from automobiles and its elasticity, the economically optimum degree of dismantling, the effect of changing technology in transportation and processing in scrap supply, the effect of labor costs and secondary materials prices on auto dismantling profits, variations in dismantling profits with the nonferrous impurities left in the hulk, and the amount of residuals formed and the cost of reducing their discharge.

In chapter 7 the various aspects of the study, both qualitative and quantitative, are brought together to give a coherent picture of the industry, its mode of operation, and its problems. Finally, chapter 8 summarizes the discussion and provides an overall perspective on the steel scrap industry and related policy issues.[7]

---

[7] The models developed are of interest to most readers from the standpoint of the conclusions to which they lead. Some readers, however, may be doing research in the steel scrap industry or in ferrous material recycling and may want extensive documentation. This is available for both models in a doctoral dissertation, "A Regional Model of the Steel Scrap Processing Sector of the Economy," by James W. Sawyer, Jr. Copies of the dissertation are available from University Microfilms, Ann Arbor, Michigan.

1

Ferrous Solid Residuals

TYPES OF RESIDUALS

Society derives rich benefits from the use of ferrous materials. Associated with these social gains, however, are social costs arising from some of the residuals which are waste products of the manufacture, use, and disposal of ferrous materials. Figure 1-1 shows the flow of activities and materials in these processes and emphasizes the various recycling loops and the production of residuals (unpriced waste products) in each step in the sequence.

Some residuals, such as water vapor produced in the combustion of fuel, are harmless. Others, however, impose costs on society in one way or another: sulfur dioxide and other gases which are a by-product of steel production are not only unpleasant but also probably associated with increased morbidity and mortality rates; the particulate matter produced in both steel production and scrap processing operations produces a physically dirty environment, thereby increasing cleaning costs and decreasing property values. It may also be associated with increased morbidity and mortality rates.

The social costs that occur as unwanted side effects of industrial operations are of great importance, for they must be taken into account in determining optimum production levels. This is no easy task when recycling is involved, for, as Spofford[1] points out, the private market system fails to allocate common property resources (air, water, land) efficiently among all users. These are the very resources that are used for disposal of residuals, but at present the cost of disposal is largely borne by the general public in the form of lowered environmental

[1] W. O. Spofford, Jr., "Solid Residuals Management, Some Economic Considerations," *Natural Resources Journal*, vol. 11 (1971), pp. 561–589.

1

quality. Thus the private market optimum does not necessarily conform to the social optimum.

Some residuals or some portions of residuals have the potential of being recycled at low net cost. An excellent example of such a residual is the particulate matter formed during the production of pig iron in a blast furnace. These particulates are mostly iron oxide. They have a high density, thus allowing for ready separation from the accompanying gas stream. But more importantly, since they contain iron, the collected particulates can serve as one of the feedstocks for the blast furnace. Thus residuals containing a large amount of iron and steel are of particular interest and receive special emphasis in figure 1-1.

There are also residuals that present specific problems because of their location. Abandoned vehicles are examples of this type of residual. Accumulating automobiles, whether scattered at random on the landscape or gathered together in the salvage yard, may impose costs on society in that they may detract from the potential natural beauty of the environment.

Residuals are a normal consequence of the production of steel scrap. The extent of this residual production has never been seriously studied, but it is common knowledge among people familiar with the scrap industry that significant amounts of solid residuals are formed in the dismantling of automobiles and their conversion to processed scrap. For example, the tires are always removed and disposed of in some way. Moreover, the newest and most advanced device for converting a dismantled automobile into usable processed scrap, the shredder, produces large amounts of airborne particulates and solid waste, and requires substantial energy inputs. In addition, the processes that convert steel scrap to useful steel produce residuals also.

Recycling versus Disposal

The question of interest here is whether the sum of all the costs, both private and social, associated with the usage of a given quantity of steel is less if the final product is processed to obtain reusable material or less if the steel object is disposed of as solid residuals after its useful life is over. While the answer intuitively seems to be the former, a detailed analysis of the problem is required to assure us that this is indeed correct.

Such a comparative analysis of "total systems" to produce a given final output might result in different answers, depending on circumstances. Consider just one of the many predominantly steel objects currently in use, the office safe. Scrap dealers refuse to purchase safes,

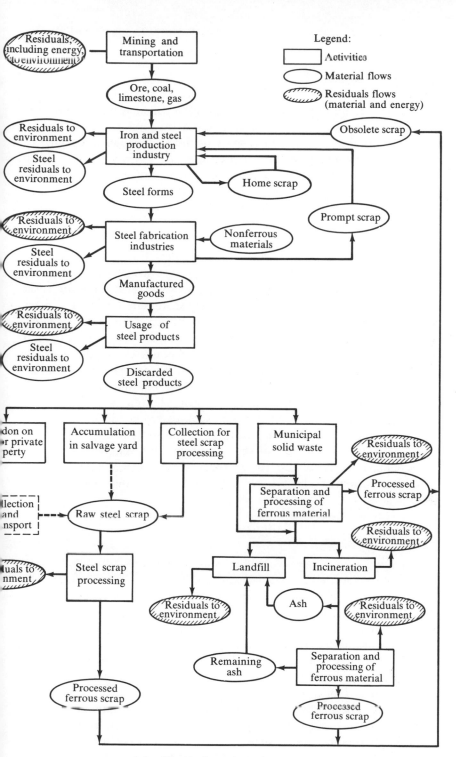

FIGURE 1-1. The steel supply system.

or even to accept them at no charge, because an office safe is usually made of a sandwich of steel and concrete. This design makes the recovery of steel so costly as to be unprofitable. This suggests that whether or not an object should be recycled will depend on the total inputs necessary for utilizing the residual as a source of raw material. The same problem exists with respect to the total inputs necessary to use "virgin" raw materials, that is, iron ore.

A second example furnishes yet another perspective on the problem. If an automobile ends its useful life near a large city with a demand for steel scrap, such as Philadelphia, there will be: (a) large numbers of other automobiles in the immediate vicinity, many of which will also be ending their useful life; and (b) low transportation costs associated with collecting the obsolete automobiles, transporting them to a processing center, and then taking the processed material to a scrap consumer. By contrast, automobiles ending their useful life in rural New Mexico are few in number and widely scattered. This makes them costly to collect and transport to the nearest scrap processing center, Albuquerque. In addition, while there is a market for scrap within a few miles of Philadelphia, the steel scrap market nearest to Albuquerque is El Paso, Texas, some 250 miles away. Therefore, the scrap product transportation costs are high. Thus it would be less than surprising if a detailed analysis of the steel scrap problem showed that the answer to the question of whether the benefits of recycling exceed the costs depends, not only on the characteristics of the used steel object under consideration (as in the case of the office safe), but also on its location at the end of its useful life (as in the case of the automobile in the New Mexico countryside).

TYPES OF SCRAP

This study is concerned with what is usually termed "obsolete" scrap, or sometimes "post-consumer" scrap, as opposed to "home" scrap and "prompt" scrap, because it is post-consumer scrap that is of most concern to society. Home scrap refers to the steel scrap that is an unavoidable nonproduct output of the steelmaking operation. For example, in the production of steel sheet, the rough edges of the sheet must be trimmed; this trim is immediately recycled in the mill to produce more steel. Prompt scrap refers to the steel that is a nonproduct output of steel fabricating operations. For example, in the fabrication of an automobile fender from steel sheet, the excess material must be trimmed off, and this trim is transported back to the steel mill for recycling to produce more steel. It is relatively easy for steel companies to recycle home and prompt scrap at a profit, since their metal content is known and large quantities are generated in a single location. As a result, home and prompt scrap impose small social costs (externalities) on society. Post-consumer, or obsolete, scrap often imposes serious costs on society, hence it should receive the most careful scrutiny. Figure 1-2 clarifies the nomenclature employed for home, prompt, and obsolete scrap.

The value of scrap, as with any raw material, is most affected by its location, quantity, and quality. As Bower[2] points out, in processing residuals, it is most desirable to have a large mass of high-quality material close to the source of production or market. The relevance of these points to ferrous scrap consumption is amply demonstrated by an examination of the relative magnitude of scrap flows, by source, in the ferrous materials industry. Two studies by Battelle Memorial Institute, one in 1957[3] and one in 1972,[4] have furnished sufficient information to allow an approximate calculation of usage of scrap, by source, in the ferrous materials industry. The Commerce Department has used the information obtained by Battelle in the 1955 study to calculate scrap flows, by source, as a percentage of total scrap flows, and has also supplied information on the total amount of scrap going to the ferrous materials industry, expressed as a percent by weight of the total metallic feed.[5]

Data calculated from the Commerce Department study (Business and Defense Services Administration—otherwise known as BDSA) are shown in figure 1-3 and in table 1-1 for the period 1947 through 1964. The data make it clear that (a) total scrap feed is more or less constant at about 50 percent by weight of total metallic feed; (b) home scrap and purchased scrap—which together constitute total scrap— are about 30 percent and 18 percent respectively of total metallic feed;

[2] U.S. Congress, Joint Economic Committee, *The Economics of Recycling Waste Materials*, Hearings before the Subcommittee on Fiscal Policy of the Joint Economic Committee, 92 Cong., 1 sess., 1971, see p. 120.

[3] Battelle Memorial Institute, *A Survey and Analysis of the Supply and Availability of Obsolete Iron and Steel Scrap*, Report to the Business and Defense Services Administration, U.S. Department of Commerce (Battelle Memorial Institute, 1957).

[4] W. J. Regan, R. W. James, and T. J. McLeer, *Final Report on Identification of Opportunities for Increased Recycling of Ferrous Solid Waste*, Report by the Battelle Memorial Institute to the Scrap Metal Research and Education Foundation of the Institute of Scrap Iron and Steel, Inc. (Institute of Scrap Iron and Steel, Inc., 1972).

[5] U.S. Department of Commerce, Business and Defense Services Administration, *Iron and Steel Scrap Consumption Problems* (Government Printing Office, Washington, D.C., 1966). See p. 46, Table A-4 for the relevant data in this report.

For an extension to 1968 of figures calculated by the same technique, see Arsen Darnay and William E. Franklin, *Salvage Markets for Materials in Municipal Solid Waste* (U.S. Environmental Protection Agency, 1972), p. 58-11. In light of the 1972 Battelle report by Regan *et al.*, these figures seem superannuated.

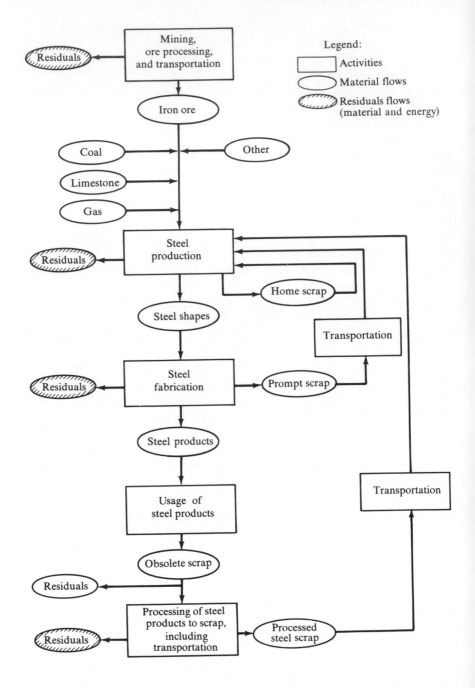

FIGURE 1-2.   Simplified flow diagram of steel supply system showing the major recycle loops.

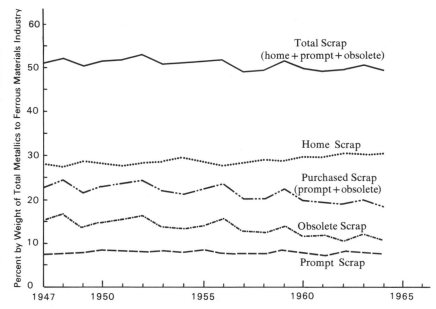

FIGURE 1-3. Scrap as a weight percentage of total metallic feed to ferrous materials industry broken down by scrap source. Department of Commerce estimate (see note 5).

(c) the home scrap portion of total metallic feed is increasing, the purchased scrap decreasing; (d) prompt scrap and obsolete scrap—which together constitute purchased scrap—are about 18 percent of the total metallic feed, with prompt scrap retaining a more or less constant percentage of the total, and obsolete being used at a lower rate at the end of the period than at the beginning (expressed as a percentage of total metallic feed); (e) in the 1960–1964 period, obsolete scrap constituted 10–12 percent by weight of the total metallic feed to the ferrous materials industry.

In 1972 Battelle completed a second major study of the steel scrap industry and in light of their new findings reported that obsolete scrap as a percentage of total purchased scrap was probably on the order of 40 percent of total purchased scrap, as compared with the 60 percent range figures previously reported (see table 1-1). The implications of Battelle's revised estimates are shown in figure 1-4 and table 1-2. Data are shown only for those years compiled by Battelle. The revised figures lead to nearly the same conclusions as the earlier work, but now obsolete scrap seems to be 6 to 8 percent by weight of total metallic feed to the ferrous materials industry.

These figures (from both present and earlier estimates) call for careful examination of the problems in their calculations, thereby removing

TABLE 1-1.   Iron and Steel Scrap Consumption as Percent by Weight of
Total Metallics to Ferrous Materials Industry

Date	Total scrap[a]	Home scrap	Purchased scrap (Prompt and obsolete)	Prompt scrap	Obsolete scrap	Obsolete as % of purchased scrap
1947	51.1	28.2	22.9	7.6	15.3	66.7
1948	52.0	27.6	24.4	7.8	16.6	68.0
1949	50.4	28.7	21.7	8.0	13.7	63.1
1950	51.5	28.2	23.3	8.4	14.8	63.6
1951	51.8	27.9	23.9	8.3	15.6	65.3
1952	52.9	28.4	24.5	8.1	16.4	67.0
1953	50.8	28.8	22.0	8.3	13.7	62.2
1954	51.1	29.6	21.5	8.1	13.4	63.3
1955	51.3	28.8	22.5	8.5	14.0	62.2
1956	51.7	28.1	23.6	7.8	15.8	67.0
1957	49.1	28.8	20.3	7.6	12.7	62.7
1958	49.6	29.3	20.3	7.7	12.6	62.0
1959	51.7	29.2	22.5	8.5	14.1	62.7
1960	49.9	30.1	19.8	8.0	11.8	59.6
1961	49.4	29.9	19.5	7.4	12.0	61.5
1962	49.8	30.7	19.1	8.2	10.8	56.5
1963	50.7	30.5	20.2	8.1	12.1	60.0
1964	49.5	30.7	18.8	7.9	10.8	57.4

[a] From U.S. Department of Commerce, Business and Defense Services Administration, *Iron and Steel Scrap Consumption Problems* (Washington, D.C.: Government Printing Office, 1966), p. 48.

from them that aura of certainty that the printed word only too often assumes. The 1972 Battelle report expresses caution, but finds basically no reason to doubt the new results:

It is cautioned that these figures are only an approximation. All prompt industrial scrap is not recycled, although the amount not recycled is probably less than 10 percent. The same is true of home scrap. Some losses occur. In addition, inventory changes on a year-to-year basis further distort the tonnage.

It is interesting to note that these estimates are in sharp contrast to the relative importance of prompt industrial and obsolete scrap indicated in previous studies. The BDSA study estimated prompt industrial and obsolete at 16 percent and 24 percent respectively of total scrap. These estimates . . . reverse the order. While recognizing these estimates as only calculated, they are generally confirmed by the extensive survey conducted in conjunction with this study. The survey indicated that 46 percent of the establishments contacted received over 50 percent of their scrap volume from industrial sources; an additional 25 percent received 26–50 percent of their raw material from industrial sources. While obviously some industrial source material could be considered obsolete, e.g., machinery, buildings, etc., most of it would be prompt industrial, . . .

While total scrap consumption therefore has maintained a relatively stable

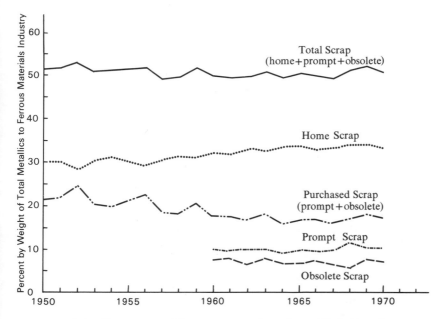

FIGURE 1-4. Scrap as a weight percentage of total metallic feed to ferrous materials industry broken down by scrap source. Revised estimate from Regan *et al.* (see note 4).

proportion of total ferrous input to iron and steelmaking, the purchased scrap portion has shown a significant decline.* During the period 1950–1956, purchased scrap accounted for 42 percent of the total scrap consumed versus 33.5 percent for the period 1964–1970. Thus, while total steel production increased 35 percent over the period 1950–1979, and total scrap consumption increased 30 percent, purchased scrap increased only 8 percent. . . .

The decline in the purchased scrap proportion of total scrap consumption can be traced to the increased generation of home scrap over this period. Mills, in essence, became greater suppliers of scrap to themselves. Yield, the amount of finished steel shipments from ingot production, provides one measure of this increased home scrap generation. While inventory shifts, shipping patterns, and changes in processing and product mix make this

---

* Statistics are not currently available on the actual amount of purchased and produced scrap consumed: only total consumption, total receipts from all sources, production, shipments, and inventories. It has been assumed for purposes of this analysis that purchased scrap = receipts — shipments. It is recognized that this calculation does not insure complete accuracy relative to consumption, due to inventory and other changes. However, the assumption that total purchased and produced approximate consumption appears valid; since 1950, the deviation between consumption and total as derived has exceeded 2 percent on only two occasions, both during inventory build-up.

TABLE 1-2.   Iron and Steel Scrap Consumption as Percent by Weight of
Total Metallics to Ferrous Materials Industry, Revised Estimate

Date	Total scrap[a]	Home scrap[b]	Purchased scrap[b] (Prompt and obsolete)	Prompt scrap[b]	Obsolete scrap[b]	Obsolete as % of purchased scrap
1950	51.5	30.0	21.5	—	—	—
1951	51.8	30.0	21.8	—	—	—
1952	52.9	28.4	24.5	—	—	—
1953	50.8	30.5	20.3	—	—	—
1954	51.1	31.2	19.9	—	—	—
1955	51.3	30.1	21.2	—	—	—
1956	51.7	29.3	22.4	—	—	—
1957	49.1	30.7	18.4	—	—	—
1958	49.6	31.4	18.2	—	—	—
1959	51.7	31.3	20.4	—	—	—
1960	49.9	32.3	17.6	10.1	7.5	42.6
1961	49.4	31.9	17.5	9.8	7.8	44.5
1962	49.8	33.1	16.7	10.1	6.6	39.4
1963	50.7	32.6	18.0	10.1	7.9	43.8
1964	49.5	33.5	16.0	9.2	6.7	41.8
1965	50.4	33.7	16.7	9.8	6.9	41.2
1966	50.0	33.0	17.0	9.6	7.4	43.5
1967	49.4	33.2	16.2	9.7	6.5	40.1
1968	51.2	34.0	17.2	11.4	5.7	33.2
1969	52.1	34.1	18.0	10.5	7.5	41.6
1970	50.7	33.4	17.3	10.2	7.0	40.4

[a] Data from U.S. Department of the Interior, *Bureau of Mines Minerals Yearbook*, vols. from 1950 to 1970.
[b] Data from W. J. Regan, R. W. James, and T. J. McLeer, *Final Report on Identification of Opportunities for Increased Recycling of Ferrous Solid Waste*, Report by the Battelle Memorial Institute to the Scrap Metal Research and Education Foundation of the Institute of Scrap Iron and Steel (1972), pp. 76, 134, and 135.

measure rather crude for year-to-year analysis, certain patterns do emerge over time. The lower yields taking place over the past 20 years are shown below [data are from annual statistical reports of the American Iron and Steel Institute].

Years	Calculated raw steel production (thousand net tons)	Calculated finished steel shipments (thousand net tons)	Yield (percent)
1950–1954	495,126	367,470	74.2
1955–1959	523,668	377,154	72.0
1960–1964	531,961	368,327	69.2
1965–1969	665,500	452,291	68.0

Another approach that indicates increased home scrap generation can be seen from a comparison of scrap produced by the mills and product shipments. Again, averages have been used, as year-to-year figures allow distortion of the pattern [data are from annual statistical reports of the American Iron and Steel Institute].

Years	Scrap produced (thousand net tons)	Steel shipments (thousand net tons)	Ratio: Scrap produced to steel shipments
1950–1954	160,325	367,470	.44
1955–1959	168,898	377,154	.45
1959–1964	181,924	368,327	.49
1965–1969	232,974	452,291	.52

The increased generation of home scrap has been caused by numerous factors. While processing equipment has been substantially upgraded over this period to provide better and higher yield products, the quality demands of the marketplace, increasing competition between both domestic and foreign producers, and the changing product mix toward lighter, flat rolled products from heavier sections have required increased quality control measures, resulting in lower yields from raw steel production. For example, in 1950, flat rolled products accounted for slightly over 35 percent of total steel shipments; in 1969, the flat rolled proportion had grown to 47 percent. Production of alloy and stainless steels, with lower product yields than carbon steels, has increased. Standard and line pipe, rails and accessories, plates, and semi-finished (with the exception of the recent export surge) have all shown decreases over this period [see note 4, pp. 71, 72, 134, 136, and 137].

Thus the findings have been carefully considered by the Battelle researchers and deemed well substantiated.

A strong attack on the validity of the data could nonetheless be made. There is, in fact, no way of knowing (at the present time) what percentage of purchased scrap materials consists of prompt scrap and what percentage consists of obsolete scrap. However, the percentage of metallics feed that consists of purchased scrap can be established with near certainty.[6] Both studies indicate it to have been decreasing in recent years, and to be currently about 17 or 18 percent of metallic feed. Clearly, the maximum possible consumption of obsolete scrap is currently 17–18 percent because it is simply not credible that prompt scrap is an insignificant portion of purchased scrap, as is known from both Battelle studies. In the fabrication of steel products, prompt scrap is produced in large quantities. In the 1957 Battelle study, prompt scrap generation ratios (defined as one hundred times scrap generation shipments divided by materials consumption) ranged from 4 to 50 percent, with the majority of the values being in the 15 to 30 percent range. These data are for 1954. Therefore the assumption that they still hold

---

[6] Each year the U.S. Department of the Interior publishes the *Bureau of Mines Minerals Yearbook* (in 4 volumes) and the scrap data therein is also published monthly by the Bureau of Mines. The "Iron and Steel Scrap" section of the yearbook contains a table of scrap and pig iron consumption, and scrap production, by type of ferrous materials manufacturer. The amount of purchased scrap can be readily calculated from this data.

exactly is unwarranted, but it may be safely assumed that they have not changed radically.

Thus while it is not possible to make firm estimates of the percentage of obsolete scrap in the total metallic feed going to the ferrous materials industry, it is clear that it must be far less than 17 percent. The 6–12 percent range seems reasonable, and in view of the latest Battelle study, *it would seem that the current value is closer to six than it is to twelve.*[7]

The rather extensive treatment of percent of recycling given here is intended to eliminate confusion in later analyses. Total obsolete scrap is about 40 percent of total purchased scrap feed.[8] Automobiles apparently

---

[7] It is natural to think it anomalous that, whereas 20 years ago obsolete scrap and prompt scrap were about 60 percent and 40 percent respectively of total purchased scrap, now they are about 40 percent and 60 percent respectively. However, it is not clear that this implies an error in one of the two calculations, or even that there has been a fundamental change in the modus operandi of the scrap market. The seeming anomaly may be only a reflection of an unstated and perhaps erroneous hypothesis; namely that the ratio of obsolete to prompt stays the same.

Consider a different and inherently more plausible hypothesis: that prompt scrap generation ratios stay more or less constant. If this is so, then an interesting train of logic makes the inversion of obsolete and prompt scrap production rates quite plausible. Total scrap consumption, as a percentage of total metallics feed, has stayed constant at about 50 percent by weight. Moreover, home scrap production has risen—therefore purchased scrap production has fallen. But the supply of prompt scrap (as a percentage of steel sales) has remained constant. The steel industry has consistently stated its need for high quality scrap, and prompt scrap is almost always of higher quality than obsolete scrap. Therefore prompt scrap will be purchased preferentially to obsolete scrap. Thus whereas at one time obsolete scrap sales exceeded prompt scrap sales, as purchased scrap sales continue to decline and prompt scrap sales stay constant, obsolete scrap sales must continue to decline. The time must inevitably come when prompt scrap sales will exceed obsolete scrap sales. So there is not necessarily a reason to think that there is some contradiction between the findings of the two Battelle reports.

If this is true, why is it not indicated in figures 1-1 and 1-2? Simply because these two figures are calculated on the assumption that the ratios of obsolete to prompt are a constant. In the light of the present discussion, this assumption seems rather tenuous. The data in tables 1-1 and 1-2 add considerable plausibility to the alternative hypothesis presented here. The prompt scrap feed was 7–8.5 percent by weight in the first study (in which the obsolete to prompt ratio was about 60:40), and about 9–10 percent by weight in the second Battelle study (in which the obsolete to prompt ratio was about 40:60). This suggests that in fact, prompt scrap to total metallics feed ratios have stayed relatively constant. Therefore, since purchased scrap to total metallics ratios have decreased considerably, obsolete scrap to prompt scrap ratios would be expected to decrease from greater than one to less than one.

[8] It is difficult to use industry classifications to estimate the rate of formation of raw obsolete scrap. No figures are compiled by either government or industry, and the validity of assuming that scrap formation rates are essentially in the same industrial order (in terms of magnitude) as current steel purchasing rates is confounded by the facts that: (a) growth rates in some industries are higher than in others; and (b) lifetimes of steel objects vary widely. Steel purchases for 1970 by industry are shown below in order of size, and give some idea of the relative

make up 50 to 60 percent of this obsolete scrap supply. Thus great care must be exercised in discussing elasticities of supply. If this is kept in mind, it will reduce the possibility of misinterpreting the results of this analysis.

For all this attention to scrap flows, and for all their importance, it is erroneous to conclude that a post-consumer scrap feed rate of 6 to 8 percent of total metallics is low, optimum, or high. As Spofford points out,[9] determining the optimal reuse ratio is not a simple matter. Because of residuals handling and disposal costs, the optimal reuse ratio for the private market will generally be less than the social optimum unless all costs are internalized. Determination of the socially optimal reuse ratio requires hard data on methods of handling and disposal of residuals; reuse systems; production processes; alternative factor inputs to pro-

---

quantities of a particular industry's product in the obsolete scrap stream. See American Iron and Steel Institute, *Annual Statistical Report, 1971* (and previous years) (American Iron and Steel Institute, 1972).

Industry	1970 Purchases in 000's of net tons
Automotive	14,475
Construction	10,565
Containers, packages, and shipping materials	7,775
Industrial machinery, equipment, and tools	5,169
Construction products	4,440
Rail transportation	3,097
Electrical equipment	2,694
Appliances, utensils, and cutlery	2,160
Other domestic and commercial equipment	1,778

The problems of using such a list for scrap estimations can be seen in three specific examples: First, approximately 6 million gross tons of scrap steel were produced from automobiles in 1970. Second, the containers–packages–shipping materials classification is made up of mostly short lifetime products such as cans. Therefore, this industry might reasonably be expected to produce perhaps 5 million gross tons per year of obsolete scrap, very little of which is recycled. Third, while steel purchases for rail transportation are relatively low, the product lifetimes are high (perhaps 35–50 years). Hence the scrap being made from railroad industry material has as its source the equipment purchased during the golden age of rail-roading, so that railroad scrap availability is much greater than might be suggested by the list. Railroad scrap sales in 1970 were 2–3 million net tons.

Those who are researching steel scrap should be aware of the work of Darnay and Franklin, who report figures for source of obsolete scrap as a percent of the total obsolete scrap. They indicate that auto wreckers (in 1959) accounted for only about 13 percent by weight of total obsolete scrap, a value that conflicts sharply with Stone's estimate for 1968 (see note 10) of about 33 percent. See Darnay and Franklin, *Salvage Markets*, table 36, p. 58-14. The value of 50–60 percent used here seems more realistic in view of the small size of the total obsolete scrap market and the reatively large size of the auto scrap market.

[9] Spofford, "Solid Residuals Management."

duction; residuals generation associated with each production process; and finally the market and nonmarket externalities of production, reuse, and disposal.

This information does not exist to date and its absence precludes an analysis of the social, political, and institutional constraints operating on an optimal economic system. Thus, there is no basis for stating that a particular feed rate is low or optimum. At present no objective judgment can be made.

AUTOMOBILE-DERIVED SCRAP

This study concentrates on autos for three reasons. First, automobiles represent the largest single source of post-consumer steel scrap.[10] An idea of the importance automobile-derived scrap has for the steel industry can be gained from figure 1-5. Only about 6–12 percent of the

[10] Ralph Stone and Co., Inc., *Copper Control in Vehicular Scrap*, Contract No. 14-09-0070-382, for Bureau of Mines (U.S. Department of the Interior, March 1968), see especially p. 43.

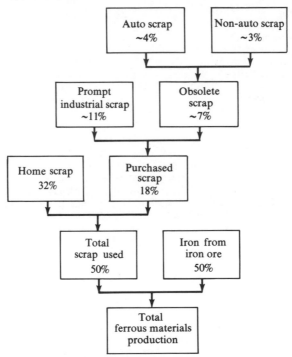

FIGURE 1-5. Origin of materials used in making ferrous materials. All percentage values given are percentages of total ferrous feed to steel production. Data are for 1970.

raw material for ferrous materials production is obsolete, or post-consumer, steel scrap. Thirty to 40 percent of this obsolete steel scrap is derived from automobiles. Second, discarded automobiles are the most visible example of once-useful steel objects which can produce disamenities after use. Obsolete automobiles that are not buried or processed into steel scrap often are eyesores. Third, more information is available on the processing of automobiles into a valuable raw material than on any other post-consumer raw steel scrap material.

2

A Qualitative Introduction to the Ferrous Scrap Industry

THE GENERATION OF RAW SCRAP

When an automobile has ended its useful life, it is removed from registration, or deregistered.[1] While the auto industry has been extensively studied and researched, studies devoted to deregistered automobiles are less common and usually have sparse technical content. They consist mostly of government pamphlets and government-sponsored studies,[2] a few semitechnical articles in various trade journals, such as

[1] The term deregistration is used in this study to replace the awkward, but more common phrase, "removal from registration." See Motor Vehicle Manufacturers Association of the U.S., Inc., *1971 Automobile Facts and Figures*, and *1972 Automobile Facts and Figures* (Motor Vehicle Manufacturers Association of the U.S., Inc., 1971, 1972).

[2] See Battelle Memorial Institute, *A Survey and Analysis of the Supply and Availability of Obsolete Iron and Steel Scrap*, Report to the Business and Defense Services Administration, Department of Commerce (Battelle Memorial Institute, 1957); R. S. Berry and M. F. Fels, *The Production and Consumption of Automobiles (An Energy Analysis of the Manufacture, Discard and Reuse of the Automobile and its Component Materials)*, Report to the Illinois Institute for Environmental Quality (Institute for Environmental Quality, 1972); W. J. Regan, R. W. James, and T. J. McLeer, *Final Report on Identification of Opportunities for Increased Recycling of Ferrous Solid Waste*, Report by the Battelle Memorial Institute to the Scrap Metal Research and Education Foundation of the Institute of Scrap Iron and Steel, Inc., (Institute of Scrap Iron and Steel, Inc., 1971); Ralph J. Stone, *Copper Control in Vehicular Scrap*, Report to the U.S. Department of the Interior, Bureau of Mines, Contract No. 14-09-0070-382 (Ralph J. Stone and Co., Inc., 1968); Ralph J. Stone, *Resource Reclamation: Yard Efficiency, A Preliminary Study of Scrapping Processes and Site Planning*, Report to the U.S. Department of the Interior, Bureau of Mines, Grant No. GO 180529 (SWD-20) (Ralph J. Stone and Co., Inc., 1969); U.S. Congress, Joint Economic Committee, *The Economics of Recycling Waste Materials*, Hearings before the Subcommittee on Fiscal Policy of the Joint Economic Committee, 92 Cong., 1 sess., 1971; U.S.

Iron Age and *Waste Age*, and, to date, three doctoral dissertations,[3] one by Plater-Zyberk, one by Adams, and one by Sawyer.[4]

To clarify discussion, the following definitions are given: an automobile that has been taken out of registration will be referred to as an obsolete automobile or a deregistered automobile. A deregistered automobile may have a part removed for sale as a replacement part, this process being referred to as auto salvaging; a deregistered automobile may have a part removed either for sale as scrap metal or because that part must be removed as preparation for final scrap processing, this process being referred to as auto dismantling. The word "hulk" or the words "auto hulk" will be used to denote a dismantled automobile; hulk processing will be used to denote the processing of hulks into salable processed scrap; and processed scrap will be used to denote the product of the hulk processor's operations. Businesses that are engaged primarily in dismantling autos to recover salvageable parts will be referred

---

Department of Commerce, Business and Defense Services Administration, *Iron and Steel Scrap Consumption Problems* (Government Printing Office, 1966); U.S. Department of Health, Education and Welfare, Public Health Service, Bureau of Solid Waste Management, *Automobile Scrapping Process and Needs for Maryland* (Government Printing Office, 1970); U.S. Department of Health, Education and Welfare, Public Health Service, Bureau of Solid Waste Management, *Dismantling Railroad Freight Cars*, by Dale M. Butler and W. M. Graham, 1969; U.S. Department of the Interior, Bureau of Mines, *Automobile Disposal, A National Problem*, 1967; U.S. Department of the Interior, Bureau of Mines, *Construction and Testing of a Junk Auto Incinerator*, by C. J. Chindgren, K. C. Dean, and J. W. Sterner, Bureau of Mines Solid Waste Research Program, Technical Progress Report 21, 1970; U.S. Department of the Interior, Bureau of Mines, *Dismantling a Typical Junk Automobile to Produce Quality Scrap*, Bureau of Mines Report of Investigations 7350, 1969; U.S. Department of the Interior, Bureau of Mines, *Preliminary Separation of Metals and Non-Metals from Urban Refuse*, by K. C. Dean, C. J. Chindgren, and LeRoy Peterson, Bureau of Mines Solid Waste Research Program, Technical Progress Report 34, 1971; U.S. Department of the Interior, Bureau of Mines, *Recovery of the Non-Ferrous Metals from Auto Shredder Rejects by Air Classification*, by C. J. Chindgren, K. C. Dean, and LeRoy Peterson, Bureau of Mines Solid Waste Research Program, Technical Progress Report 31, 1971; U.S. Department of the Interior, Bureau of Mines, *Removal of Non-Ferrous Metals from Synthetic Automobile Scrap on Heating in a Rotary Kiln*, by G. W. Elger, W. L. Hunter, and C. E. Armantrout, Bureau of Mines Report of Investigations 7210, 1968.

[3] There are also at least two interesting master's theses on steel scrap, one by Oberman (M. A. Oberman, "Analysis of a Transition in the Scrap Iron and Steel Industry," unpublished M.B.A. thesis, Northwestern University, 1966) and one by Raidy (Peter James Raidy, "The Pricing Environment of Scrap Iron and Steel," unpublished master's thesis, University of Pennsylvania, 1957).

[4] See R. Plater-Zyberk, "The Economics of Ferrous Scrap Recycling," unpublished Ph.D. thesis, Drexel University, Philadelphia, 1972, and R. L. Adams, "An Economic Analysis of the Junk Automobile Problem," unpublished Ph.D. dissertation, University of Illinois, 1972. Adams' work was done under the auspices of the U.S. Bureau of Mines and has been published by the U.S. Government Printing Office, Washington, D.C. (1973).

to as auto salvagers; businesses that are engaged primarily in dismantling autos to produce hulks as the raw material for processors will be referred to as small scrap dealers or dismantlers; businesses that are engaged primarily in transforming hulks into processed scrap material will be referred to as large-scale scrap processors. There is an overlap among these businesses. For example, some small scrap dealers have equipment with which they can convert hulks into processed scrap. In this model, however, hulk processing is assumed to be totally separated from automobile dismantling. Also, for purposes of modeling, the dismantling portion of an auto salvager's business is assumed to be totally separated from the salvage portion. Dismantling by an auto salvager will be treated exactly the same as dismantling by an auto dismantler.

The disposition of automobiles after deregistration is presented most simply in flow chart form. Figure 2-1 shows automobile movements up to the hulk processor; figure 2-2 shows the possible sequence of modifications by the hulk processor.

After automobiles are manufactured, they are used by consumers for varying lengths of time, after which they are deregistered and become a legitimate source of scrap (figure 2-1).[5] Following deregistration, the obsolete auto can either be disposed of by socially acceptable means or abandoned. In either case, there is a transportation step. If the car is not abandoned and is in operating order, the owner will probably drive it to a small scrap dealer or salvager. If not abandoned, but not in operating order, the owner will ask a scrap dealer or salvager to tow it away. If abandoned, it is usually identified by the police or sanitation department as being abandoned (after some time). In this case the city will tow it to a scrap dealer or salvager or, in many cases, a dealer who has a contract with the city to handle all abandoned cars will be notified and he will tow it to his yard.

The automobile body (or what remains of it) is dismantled by an auto salvage company or a small scrap dealer. If a salvager does the

___

[5] Many problems, primarily legal, in the disposal and abandonment of cars arise from their lack of value as raw material. Our research did not concern itself with these problems. Relevant references are mostly governmental studies: see Regan, et al., *Final Report on Identification of Opportunities*; U.S. Congress, Senate Committee on Public Works, *Disposal of Junked and Abandoned Motor Vehicles*, Hearings before the Subcommittee on Air and Water Pollution of the Committee on Public Works, Senate, on S. 4197 and S. 4204, 91 Cong., 2 sess., 1970; U.S. Department of Commerce, Business and Defense Services Administration, *Motor Vehicle Abandonment in U.S. Urban Areas*, 1967; U.S. Department of Health, Education and Welfare, *Automobile Scrapping Process*; U.S. Department of the Interior, *Automobile Disposal*, 1967. It seems clear that the legal system could be reformed to make the disposition of abandoned cars a simpler process. It is also clear that a thorough economic/legal study of the auto salvage business would be valuable, since these businesses apparently have a large inventory of auto hulks which create an aesthetic problem. See U.S. Department of the Interior, *Automobile Disposal*, 1967.

work, he may well remove some parts, such as a fender, wheel, or set of hubcaps, for sale to other automobile owners. This stage of dismantling is not pertinent to a study of the scrapping process. Only the final dismantling stages are of interest here. In these final stages, the radiator, battery, engine, tires, and gas tank are removed because the hulk processor demands their removal. These parts and others may be removed if either they or the metals from which they are made can be removed and sold at a profit as secondary metals.

Following dismantling, the hulks are shipped to hulk processors (bottom of figure 2-1, top of figure 2-2) who use large-scale, capital-

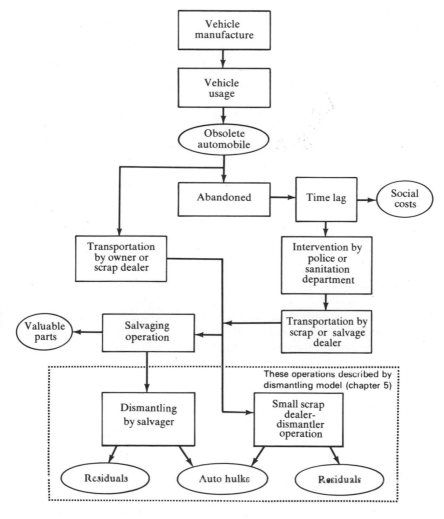

FIGURE 2-1. Flowsheet for automobile usage and scrapped automobile handling and disposal.

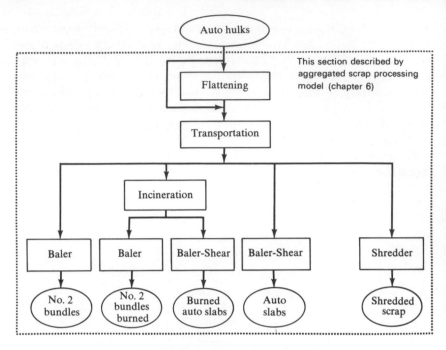

FIGURE 2-2.   Hulk processing system flow diagram.

intensive equipment to transform them into salable scrap. Hulks may be shipped individually, as a group of unflattened hulks, or as a group of flattened hulks. The method employed is related to the number of hulks the dismantler has available for shipment at the time, the availability of flattening equipment, and the distance from the dismantling location to the scrap processor. If shipping distances are much over 15 miles, the most economical way to move a significant number of hulks is by flattening and shipping them as a group. Flattening allows up to forty cars to be shipped on a truck at one time, but in the instances observed in the course of the study, a truckload usually consisted of about fifteen to twenty-five flattened hulks.

SCRAP PROCESSING EQUIPMENT

Figure 2-2 indicates the various ways hulks can be processed, all of which will be discussed below. There are four types of capital-intensive methods commonly used in converting raw material into steel scrap. These are incineration, baling, shearing, and shredding.

Incineration is still used by some scrap metal dealers to remove the readily oxidizable (largely organic) material from the metal. The two most common incinerators are those that burn the rugs, seats, paint, and wire insulation from automobiles, and those specially designed to burn insulation from wires. Only the first type of incinerator is of concern in this study. Auto hulk incinerators are relatively simple devices. They usually hold two to twelve hulks at a time. The hulks are placed on steel cars (of the railroad type, but smaller), some flammable material such as kerosene or fuel oil is poured over them, and the hulk-laden cars are wheeled into the incinerator. Burning usually takes from 30 to 45 minutes. In order to reduce particulate emissions, the incinerator off-gases are run through an afterburner. Burning is essentially complete, the hulk containing almost no organic material after the incineration step.

Open burning of auto hulks was a widely practiced substitute for incineration prior to the declaration by local governments that the amounts of particulates produced were not tolerable. In most areas of the country there is now a total ban on open burning.

The baler uses hydraulic rams to compress crushable steel objects of assorted sizes and shapes into bales (commonly called "bundles" in the trade). These bundles are rectangular parallelepipeds with densities on the order of 100–200 pounds per cubic foot. Balers come in a range of sizes and produce bundles ranging in size from 1 foot on each side to those measuring 2 by 3 by 5 feet, and weighing about 2½ tons. Balers can be used to process a large variety of residual steel products. They cannot be used for processing such items as cable (springy materials), cast iron (brittle material), or very thick material (greater than ¼ to ½ inch).

There are two types of shears or shearing equipment, the newer of which is the guillotine shear. Its name derives from the fact that the shear blade and the framework within which it is placed resemble a guillotine. The blade is powered hydraulically and has the capability, in a large unit, of cutting through a solid steel cylinder 6 inches in diameter. It can cut up to 150,000 to 200,000 tons of scrap a year.[6] Before 1956, an alligator shear with a stationary lower jaw was used. This device required two men to operate it, in addition to the feeders, and used a significant amount of hand labor. Conveyors for automatically feeding the scrap into the shear have increased its efficiency and the machine is still used today in smaller scrap processing operations.[7]

A shear is sometimes referred to as a baler-shear. In these cases a feedbox is associated with the shear and the feed is partially compressed

[6] See M. A. Oberman, "Analysis of a Transition in the Scrap Iron and Steel Industry," pp. 55–59.
[7] *Ibid.*

into the shape of a log in the feedbox. The log is then fed into the shear and cut up into blocks of semicompressed steel in the shape of small pillows,[8] and the finished material is usually referred to as slabs, or auto slabs.

The most recently developed of all the scrap processes is shredding. Entire automobiles from which the tires, gas tanks, radiators, engines, and (usually) seats have been removed are fed into a hammer mill (grinder).[9] The mill literally shreds the automobile into fist-size pieces of primarily steel material. The product is then passed through a series of air knives and magnetic separators. The air knives remove non-metallic debris. The magnetic separators separate the ferrous from the nonferrous (more precisely the magnetic from the nonmagnetic) fractions, thereby ensuring both a low contamination level product and a nonferrous product stream which may be sold at a profit. To reduce particulate emissions, shredders nearly always have cyclone separators to remove the dust particles from the air streams. In addition, some (though only a small fraction) have devices for blanketing the hammer mill with inert gas to minimize the explosion hazard.[10] The shredder is of particular interest to the student of the recycling problem because of all the machines that scrap processors use, it is the only mechanical process (with its associated equipment) capable of removing some of the nonferrous impurities.

[8] In other words, in a baler-shear, the feed is baled (that is, slightly compressed) and then sheared.

[9] The words shredder or grinder, as used here, denote the entire shredder system, including magnetic and organic separation with air knives, rather than just a hammer mill portion of the process.

[10] The explosion hazard in a shredder is due in rare cases to the failure of the dismantler to remove the gasoline tank. In most cases, however, explosions occur because, even though the gas tank has been removed, the liquid organic material in the hulk, such as the oil in the differential or the hydraulic fluid in an automatic transmission, is broken up into fine droplets during shredding, and these have the potential for ignition. Once ignited, they burn so rapidly as to form an explosion.

3

Processed Ferrous Scrap Grades and Steel Scrap Quality

DEFINITIONAL PROBLEMS IN GRADING SCRAP

In the most recent presentation of ferrous scrap quality definitions, issued by the Institute of Scrap Iron and Steel (ISIS) in 1972,[1] 72 grades of processed ferrous scrap are listed (in addition to a long list of processed railroad scrap grades and processed alloy scrap grades). The nomenclature of the ferrous scrap industry is at first bewildering. The apparent complexity is due not only to the large number of grades of scrap but also to communication difficulties which naturally arise among some 2,000 geographically dispersed and relatively small businessmen and their customers.[2] Therefore, a discussion of the scrap industry tends to be provincial unless a special effort is made to overcome the definitional difficulties. Second, the variety of definitions sets up a communication barrier between the people in the scrap business and researchers and policy makers that can only be overcome by serious intellectual efforts.

In this study an attempt has been made to surmount these obstacles and to point them out for future researchers in such a way as to make

[1] See Institute of Scrap Iron and Steel, *Specifications* (Institute of Scrap Iron and Steel, 1971).

[2] This very sentence is an example of a communications problem faced by the student. What are customers? To the layman, they are the buyers of goods. To the scrap dealer, they are the sellers from whom he buys obsolete materials (which are the scrap dealer's raw materials). See M. A. Oberman, "Analysis of a Transition in the Scrap Iron and Steel Industry," unpublished master's thesis, Northwestern University, 1966, p. 43. This is such common parlance in the scrap industry that when I asked a scrap dealer (and a rather articulate dealer at that) why the suppliers were called customers, he answered with a puzzled look on his face, "What else would you call them?"

23

this material as generally valuable as possible. Trips to scrap dealers in Illinois, Michigan, Ohio, Pennsylvania, Delaware, and Virginia have provided a broad acquaintance with the industry in the northeastern part of the United States. Nonetheless, limitations of time and money did not permit nationwide travel, and it seems clear that a description of the scrap industry which is geographically generalizable must await contributions by other researchers, scrap processors, and scrap users from all areas of the country.

Processed steel scrap that is identical in physical configuration, chemical quality, density, and (perhaps) source, may be graded differently in different parts of the country. That is to say, scrap grading is location specific. For example, an obsolete steel product such as an I-beam can be processed (cut into short lengths) into scrap. In Philadelphia this scrap would sell for No. 1 Heavy Melting, but it would probably sell as Foundry Steel (which commands a higher price) in Toledo, Ohio. This is true in spite of the fact that in both cases the product might be exactly the same shape, size, and chemical composition.

It can be argued that, rather than grades being location specific, they are specified partly by end use. For example, a used I-beam being sold to a steel mill might be termed No. 1 Heavy Melting, while if the same I-beam were sold to a foundry, it would be termed Foundry Grade. While this seems to be true, judged from interviews with scrap dealers, it also seems to be true that location specificity prevails as well.[3]

The discussion of scrap grades given here is restricted to those grades that comprise automobile scrap and grades whose inclusion is essential to the understanding of the production and use of steel scrap derived from automobiles.[4]

---

[3] Personal interviews at company offices with Calvin Lieberman, Ace Steel Baling, Inc., Toledo, Ohio, December 23, 1971 and May 12, 1972.

[4] No. 1 Heavy Melting, the highest quality level scrap, is included, for example, because in the production of drawing quality steel in the basic oxygen furnace (BOF), low quality (high copper, nickel, chromium, molybdenum, and tin content) No. 2 Bundles derived from automobiles must be diluted with a large quantity of No. 1 Heavy Melting to achieve acceptable quality steels. Thus, while there is one engineering constraint on the usage of scrap in the BOF due to heat effects (30 percent scrap maximum amount usable without gas injection), there is a more severe constraint on the amount of automobile scrap that can be used (that is, 3 percent), if the automobile scrap is in the form of No. 2 Bundles and the output desired is drawing quality steel. For a detailed discussion of this problem, see the forthcoming work of W. J. Vaughan, Resources for the Future, Inc., Washington, D.C. Vaughan is developing a mathematical model of the steel industry which will predict the demand for steel scrap and will incorporate residuals production. (Numerous personal interviews, 1972.)

SCRAP GRADES AND ASSOCIATED PROCESSES

The major grades of processed scrap are No. 1 Heavy Melting Steel and No. 2 Heavy Melting Steel. These are officially defined as:[5]

No. 1 Heavy Melting Steel. Wrought iron and/or steel scrap ¼ inch and over in thickness. Individual pieces not over 60 × 24 inches (charging box size) prepared in a manner to insure compact charging.

No. 2 Heavy Melting Steel. Wrought iron and steel scrap, black and galvanized, ⅛ inch and over in thickness, charging box size to include material not suitable as No. 1 Heavy Melting Steel. Prepared in a manner to insure compact charging.

No. 2 Heavy Melting Steel.[6] Wrought iron and steel scrap, black and galvanized, maximum size 36 × 18 inches. May include all automobile scrap properly prepared.

In addition to these definitions, the use of the terms "No. 1" and "No. 2" have additional connotations. When a scrap processor refers to No. 1 he is referring to the class of *all* nonobsolete steel scrap. That is, in general the product is either home scrap or prompt scrap. When he refers to No. 2 he is referring to the class of *all* obsolete steel scrap. Moreover, No. 1 also has the connotation of cleanliness, that is, free of foreign debris, or chemically similar to home scrap, even if it is not, strictly speaking, new. Similarly, No. 2 has the connotation of contamination.

A scrap material made with balers is always termed bundled scrap. The bundles are of different grades depending on the quality of the material from which they are made. The highest quality bundle is a No. 1 Factory Bundle, which is made from homogeneous new (home or prompt) scrap steel with no paint or nonferrous elements present, except those in solid solution in the steel. Factory bundles receive a premium price because they have no contaminating elements.

There is no product in the Philadelphia area sold by the name of factory bundles. This does not mean that this quality scrap is not sold in the region. In the particular case of No. 1 Factory Bundles, while these are not sold in the Philadelphia region, there is a product termed "Budd Bundles" (named after the Budd Company, a well-known manufacturer of metal stampings in the area). These bundles have all the defined characteristics of the officially defined No. 1 Factory Bundle.

---

[5] See Institute of Scrap Iron and Steel, *Specifications*, p. 3.

[6] The confusing identical designations given for any two classifications in the ISIS specifications arise from ambiguous industry usage. The quotations given here and on the following pages are verbatim from the most definitive source of scrap grade definitions. See footnote 5.

Nevertheless, in Philadelphia this grade of scrap is sold as Budd Bundles. This is an example of the location-specific grading phenomenon mentioned above.

Next in line of quality in the family of baled products is the No. 1 Bundle, which is defined as:[7]

No. 1 Bundles. New black steel sheet scrap, clippings or skeleton scrap, compressed or hand bundled to charging box size, and weighing not less than 75 pounds per cubic foot. (Hand bundles are tightly secured for handling with a magnet.) May include Stanley balls or mandrel wound bundles or skeleton reels, tightly secured. May include chemically detinned material. May not include old auto body or fender stock. Free of metal coated, limed, vitreous enameled, and electrical sheet containing over 0.5 percent silicon.

The most common baled product is the so-called No. 2 Bundle, usually made from scrapped automobiles. The ISIS definition of this product is:[8]

No. 2 Bundles. Old black and galvanized steel sheet scrap, hydraulically compressed to charging box size and weighing not less than 75 pounds per cubic foot. May not include tin or lead-coated material or vitreous enameled material.

There are also "Burned Bundles" which are not officially defined in the ISIS specification handbook. They are, however, available for sale in the Philadelphia area, though the market is small. A "Burned Bundle" may be defined as a bundle composed of the same material as the No. 2 Bundle, but the material is burned prior to the baling step. The burning eliminates most of the organic material, i.e., rubber (hoses, etc.) or nonrubber (paint, plastic).

This study deals explicitly with automobile-derived scrap. As such, the only types of bundled scrap explicitly included in the model are No. 2 Bundles and Burned Bundles.

A shear, or more correctly a baler-shear, can be used for producing a wide variety of scrap products. Of these, only No. 2 Heavy Melting Steel and auto slabs will be discussed here. In addition, burned auto slabs are available in the Philadelphia market area, though not in large quantity. Burned auto slabs, like burned No. 2 Bundles, are not defined by the ISIS. ISIS definitions for auto slabs are:[9]

Auto Slabs.   Clean automobile slabs, cut 3 feet × 18 inches and under.
Auto Slabs.   Clean automobile slabs, cut 2 feet × 18 inches and under.

[7] See Institute of Scrap Iron and Steel, *Specifications*, pp. 4–6, 51.
[8] *Ibid.*
[9] *Ibid.*

Both grades of auto slabs are considered here as one material, as are both grades of No. 2 Heavy Melting scrap, which are defined at the beginning of this section.

The two grades produced by shredders are "Shredded Scrap" and "Shredded Scrap." These are officially defined as:[10]

Shredded Scrap. Homogeneous iron and steel scrap, magnetically separated, originating from automobiles, unprepared No. 1 and No. 2 steel, miscellaneous baling and sheet scrap. Average density 50 pounds per cubic foot.

Shredded Scrap. Homogeneous iron and steel scrap magnetically separated, originating from automobiles, unprepared No. 1 and No. 2 steel, miscellaneous baling and sheet scrap. Average density 70 pounds per cubic foot.[11]

IMPURITIES IN SCRAP

In the production of ferrous materials, manufacturers must meet certain product quality specifications. These physical property specifications are related to the impurities present in the steel. Generally, for steels that are to be rolled into very thin sheets and then formed into complex shapes, as in the manufacture of auto body panels, it is necessary to keep the steel very low in alloying metals. The essence of the scrap quality problem is that the total car contains large amounts of nonferrous metals, primarily in the form of add-on parts, such as wiring, generators, and radiators. When the car is scrapped, if it is merely compressed into a bundle, much of the alloying material will remain and be introduced into the steel furnace when the resulting bundle is charged. Unfortunately, with the exception of chromium, these impurities (copper, molybdenum, nickel, and tin) are wholly transferred from the metallic (scrap) inputs to the steel output, and are not eliminated from the steel

---

[10] *Ibid.*

[11] In an interview with a member of the ISIS committee on scrap quality definitions (personal interview with W. Guggenheim, Plant Manager, Prolerized Chicago Corp., Chicago, May 10, 1972) and in interviews with numerous shredder operators (D. Allen and S. Allen, Sam Allen and Sons, Inc., Pontiac, Mich., June 9, 1972 and May 9, 1972; C. Brandenburg and R. L. Nauert, Luria Brothers and Co., Inc., Cleveland, Ohio, April 18, 1972; A. Goldstan, Goldstan Scrap Processing Company, Reading, Pa., June 13, October and November 1972) it became clear that the explanation of the two definitions lies in the capabilities of the shredding plants already built. The less well engineered shredders do not give the operator much control over the product bulk density. By contrast, the best-engineered shredder operations can control the bulk density of the product from as low as the 50 lb./ft.[3] range up to the 110 lb./ft.[3] range. Since these top quality operations are located only in certain regions of the country, shredded product of high bulk density is not uniformly available throughout the United States. This problem of product density, while of background interest in understanding the state of the industry, is not of consequence to the operation of the model presented herein. The cost estimates are for a well-engineered, state of the art, plant.

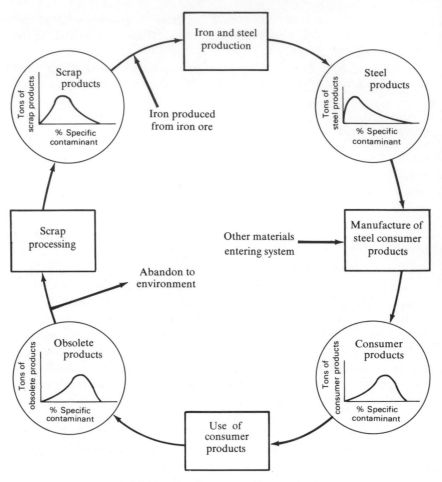

FIGURE 3-1.   Life cycle of ferrous materials.

bath by oxidation nor removed in the slag.[12] Consequently, without blending with relatively alloy-free iron or steel, it would be impossible to produce steel of auto body panel quality, using auto-hulk scrap as the furnace charge. These considerations are shown schematically in figure 3-1. In order, then, for it to be technically feasible for the annual flow of scrapped autos of given design to be absorbed as recycled ferrous inputs in the steel industry, three elements of the system must be in some rough balance:

[12] The steelmaker cannot know the exact composition of the scrap he is charging until it is melted. Therefore variability in actual quality levels within a grade inevitably results in variability in output quality. His risk of loss is reduced by reliance on customary suppliers and by allowance for a generous margin of error in choosing the charging blend.

The desired product mix and related specifications for each product
The level of impurity removal undertaken in the scrapping process
The quantity of dilution provided by the steelmaker

Beyond the questions of technical feasibility lie, of course, the problems
of economic desirability. These revolve around two major considerations: (a) the relative prices of scrap and the several inputs necessary
for the production of hot iron (especially coal, iron ore, limestone);
(b) the variability in scrap quality, even within a nominal category,
as it affects the probability of meeting the required steel specifications.
(Failure to meet specifications results in end product reclassification to
a lower quality or recycling through the furnace.[13]) What we imply
when we talk about "the scrap problem" is that the private technical and
economic decisions made by the actors involved in this system may be
different from the decisions which would be optimal from the point of
view of society as a whole. (The problems of determining socially
optimal rates are discussed in chapter 1.)

The problems of using scrap can be potentially mitigated by technology in three areas. The first area is scrap processing. An automobile,
for example, contains about 1 percent copper,[14] but through processing
this level may be reduced to some extent, though in most cases not to
the level necessary to meet the final product specifications of the steel
manufacturer.[15] Thus, because it is profitable, for direct sale, to remove
from scrapped autos a large amount of the copper introduced in manufacturing, a No. 2 Bundle contains about 0.4 to 0.5 percent copper. If
the same automobile were processed by the average shredder, the
shredded scrap would contain about 0.22 percent copper. Finally, if the
same automobile were processed by a specially designed shredder, the
copper content might well be reduced to about 0.12 percent. This will
be discussed below when the quality of shredded product is considered
in detail.

[13] Of course, the presence of nonferrous elements can be either desirable or
undesirable, depending on the grade of steel produced. For example, they may be
desirable when alloy steels, which by definition are high in these elements, must
be produced. The same elements become undesirable attributes of the scrap used
in the production of drawing quality carbon steels. Hence the difference between
the rather neutral term "residual alloy elements" and the pejorative term "tramp"
metals.
[14] See U.S. Department of the Interior, Bureau of Mines, *Automobile Disposal,
A National Problem*, 1967, p. 35. Auto body steels traditionally contain 0.05 to
0.08 percent by weight copper. [See Ralph J. Stone, *Copper Control in Vehicular
Scrap*, Report to the U.S. Department of the Interior, Bureau of Mines, Contract
No. 14-09-0070-382 (Ralph J. Stone and Co., 1968), pp. 44, 45.]
[15] This entire area has yet to receive from economists the attention it needs,
but work is forthcoming by Vaughan (see notes 4 and 20) which will deal with
the problem in significant depth. We discuss it here only in order to make clear,
in broad outline, its effect on the steel manufacturers, the scrap processors, and
their strategies for coping with it.

Copper, while it is often used as a surrogate variable by those concerned with the scrap quality problem, is only one of the five main deleterious metallic impurities.[16] Silver *et al.*[17] have studied the effects of trace metallic nonferrous contaminants on steel properties and have found copper, chromium, molybdenum, nickel, and tin to be particularly detrimental to carbon steel quality. (It should be noted that disparities between the impurity requirements for new ferrous materials and the impurity levels in scrap are not limited to automobile body steel or even deep drawing steel generally. This problem exists throughout the ferrous materials industry; for example, it occurs in ferrous casting.[18])

Silver *et al.*, after studying the individual and interactive effects of the impurities, suggest the following specifications for drawing quality (DQ) steel, the type of steel from which automobile bodies are made.

Element	Upper limit in percent by weight
Copper	0.09
Chromium	0.04
Molybdenum	0.01
Nickel	0.04
Tin	0.01
Total of all five	0.16

Thus, dilution with relatively low impurity level iron becomes a necessity for the steel manufacturer (for at least some final products) when using No. 2 Bundles as part of the charge.

The second area is the design of the automobile itself. Auto manufacturers could modify their designs so that the copper content of dismantled autos may be considerably reduced. If this were done, auto scrap from an average shredder might contain as low as 0.15 percent copper and as low as 0.09 to 0.10 percent if processed in a shredder of superior design. By mixing copper and other elements, automobile manufacturers are making it marginally more costly to recycle steel from this major source, thereby adding to the social cost of disposing

[16] Sulfur, a nonmetallic element, is also a serious impurity. Its main source is the rubber in the auto body. (Personal interview with J. Zuckerman, Zuckerman Co., Inc., Winchester, Va., June 2, 1972, and letter to J. W. Sawyer from B. Kastein, Firestone Synthetic Rubber and Latex Co., Division of Firestone Tire and Rubber Co., Akron, Ohio, October 13, 1972.) However, it is also present in the metal in the auto body.

[17] See J. Silver, P. J. Koros, L. R. Schoenberger, "The Effect of Use of Bundled Auto Scrap on Sheet Steel Quality," presented at ISIS 42nd Annual Convention, Los Angeles, 1970. Available from ISIS, Washington, D.C.

[18] For a complete table of the compositional tolerances for foundry products, see the work of the Bureau of Mines, *Automobile Disposal*, 1967, p. 26, table 2.

of obsolete automobiles. Those economists who have studied such problems[19] might advocate that a charge be levied on the nonferrous content of automobiles to repay society for the costs imposed by mixing nonferrous elements in such a way that they cannot be profitably removed.

The third area involves the technology of steel usage. Not only could the design of the different parts of an automobile be modified to reduce the presence of tramp contaminants in the scrap which may be made from it, but consideration could be given to making parts from different grades of steel where possible, thus reducing the demand for the very highest quality mild carbon steels. Low quality scrap grades may be used for products that have less severe metallurgical requirements, such as reinforcing bars, heavy structural, and heavy plate.[20]

Thus, there are three technologies relevant to the scrap impurity problem—that of the steel manufacturer, that of the manufacturer who uses steel to make consumer products—both in terms of product design and in terms of the quality of steel used to make a specific part—and that of the scrap processor.

An extensive presentation of the chemical analyses of steel scrap derived from automobiles is of value in understanding the quality problem in greater depth. A brief summary of the steel scrap analyses collected in the course of this project is presented in table 3-1. This table may be supplemented by a Battelle report[21] which is devoted specifically to the quality of No. 2 Bundles. The data in table 3-1 are relevant to the analysis of the blending problem, and of particular value in a study of the scrap business. It is apparent from the description of the steelmaker's blending problem that, in general, the higher the quality of scrap, the more desirable it is to the steel manufacturer. No. 1 Factory Bundles sell for more than Shredded Scrap, which sells for more than

[19] See John R. Hall, Russell L. Ackoff, William Finnie, Iraj Zandi, J. W. Sawyer et al., *A Systems Approach to the Problems of Solid Waste and Litter*, University of Pennsylvania, Management and Behavioral Science Center, 1971; J. M. Henderson and R. E. Quandt, *Microeconomic Theory: A Mathematical Approach* (McGraw-Hill, 1971); E. Mansfield, *Microeconomics* (W. W. Norton, 1970); G. H. K. Schenck, W. A. Lambo, and R. L. Gordon, "The Role of Secondary Materials," Paper presented at the Pennsylvania State University Forum on Technological Innovation in the Production and Utilization of Materials, National Commission on Materials Policy, University Park, Pennsylvania, June 19-21, 1972.

[20] For a detailed discussion of the steelmaking side of the "scrap problem," see W. J. Vaughan, "A Linear Programming Approach to Residuals Management in the Iron and Steel Industry," Ph.D. dissertation to be submitted to the Department of Economics, Georgetown University, Washington, D.C., 1974.

[21] See W. L. Swager, *The Measurement and Improvement of Scrap Quality* (Battelle Memorial Institute, 1960).

TABLE 3-1. Analyses of Scrap Products in Percent by Weight

	Average[a] shredded scrap	Burned[a] sheared auto scrap	No. 1[b] factory bundles	No.1[b] heavy melting	No. 2[b] dealer heavy melting	No. 2[b] dealer bundles	Ferrous metal[c] recovered from incinerator
Aluminum	ND[d]	—	—	—	—	—	—
Boron	—	—	—	—	—	—	—
Cobalt	0.009	0.015	—	—	—	—	—
Copper	0.22	0.18	0.06	0.10	0.40	0.48	0.437
Chromium	0.16	0.10	0.04	0.04	0.10	0.06	0.009
Lead	0.01	0.001	—	—	—	—	0.104
Manganese	0.151	—	—	—	—	—	0.013
Molybdenum	0.02	0.05	0.03	0.03	0.03	0.03	0.015
Nickel	0.10	0.10	0.04	0.05	0.20	0.09	0.100
Tin	0.021	0.032	0.005	0.010	0.027	0.060	0.165
Tungsten	0.004	0.01	—	—	—	—	—
Vanadium	0.010	—	—	—	—	—	—
Zinc	—	—	—	—	—	—	0.020
Carbon	0.083	—	—	—	—	—	0.034
Phosphorus	0.023	0.035	—	—	—	—	—
Silicon	0.194	0.15	—	—	—	—	—
Sulfur	0.039	0.045	0.025	0.035	0.080	0.100	0.032
% recovery[e]	97	95	97	97	89	85	—

[a] Calculated from data compiled in the course of this study from scrap processors and steel companies who prefer to remain anonymous.

[b] See C. C. Custer, "The Quality Aspects of a Cold Metal Practice vs. a Hot Metal Practice," Paper presented at the Forty-Seventh National Open Hearth and Basic Oxygen Steel Conference, AIME, April 13, 1964. Cited by W. J. Regan et al., *Final Report on Identification of Opportunities for Increased Recycling of Ferrous Solid Waste.* Report by the Battelle Memorial Institute to the Scrap Metal Research and Education Foundation of the Institute of Scrap Iron and Steel, Inc., 1971.

[c] See E. J. Ostrowski, "Recycling of Tin Free Steel Cans, Tin Cans, and Scrap from Municipal Incinerator Residue," Paper presented at the 79th General Meeting of the American Iron and Steel Institute, New York, N.Y., May 26, 1971.

[d] No data.

[e] $\% \text{ recovery} = \dfrac{\text{weight of steel}}{\text{weight of charge}} \times 100$

No. 1 Bundles, which sell for more than No. 2 Bundles.[22] Pursuing the suggested generalization—the higher the quality the more valuable the scrap—a close examination of the data on shredded scrap in table 3-1 is in order. The processes of baling and baling-shearing, for all practical purposes, do not significantly change the level of nonferrous metallic impurities in steel scrap derived from automobiles. For the shredding process this is not the case. Thus, of the scrap processing technologies available today, the shredder offers the greatest potential for improving the quality of scrap and increasing its usefulness.

In 1964 the Manufacturing Group of General Motors began a fairly extensive effort to understand the role of automobiles in scrap utilization. Their work has been reported by Uhlig.[23] Of GM's efforts, that of most relevance to this study related to impurities in shredded scrap. General Motors personnel first analyzed shredded scrap from the two largest scrap processors in the United States, Luria Brothers (a division of the Ogden Corp.) and Proler.[24] They then evaluated the technical feasibilty of making marked improvements in scrap quality. Their attention quickly focused on the process of Sam Allen and Sons in Pontiac, Michigan.[25] The Allen process involves ripping the hulks (with a machine appropriately called a "ripper"), shredding, and then, as in all shredding plants, running the material through a series of magnetic separators. The ripping operation entails literally tearing the automobile into eight or ten pieces.[26] Allen's material was being used at the Pontiac Motor Division foundry (located in Pontiac). General Motors analyzed the product and found it to be of significantly higher quality than the average shredder scrap. They then took one batch of two, the second batch serving as a control, and treated it with an additional screening and magnetic separation. Neither batch underwent any hand picking or

[22] Shredded scrap, the price of which is not listed in the commodity price lists currently obtainable in *Iron Age*, sells for a price "at least equal to the price of No. 1," in the words of nearly every shredder operator we have visited (the names of the specific processors who made this statement are withheld at their request). This fact is not a result of a purity level greater than No. 1, but rather is apparently due to its better handling properties (it flows).

The problem of validating the scrap dealer's comments with actual price data is dealt with in chapter 7, appendix A in which it is demonstrated from export data that the price of shredded scrap is essentially equivalent to the price of No. 1.

[23] See U.S. Congress, Senate Committee on Public Works, *Resource Recovery Act of 1969 (Part 3)*, Hearings before the Subcommittee on Air and Water Pollution, Senate, on S. 2005, 91 Cong., 2 sess., 1970. pp. 1658–1671.

[24] In the course of this study one plant run by each of these corporations was visited.

[25] This operation was also visited. Personal interview at the company offices of Sam Allen and Sons, Inc., Pontiac, Mich., May 9, 1972.

[26] This "ripper" is manufactured by the Ripsteel Corp. of Milwaukee, Wis., and is described in their Bulletin 67 (Martin H. Panning, Ripsteel Corp., letter to J. W. Sawyer, May 16, 1972).

sorting at the discharge end of the conveyors. Analysis of this product showed an even higher quality level than that of Allen's product. The results of the GM tests are summarized in table 3-2. Uhlig, on the basis of this, has stated that copper levels of 0.12 percent could be realistically and consistently achieved on a commercial basis by the scrap processing industry.[27]

The GM work (table 3-2) (as well as some of the analyses collected in the course of this study) indicates that substantial improvements in the quality of shredded scrap are probably possible with relatively minor design modifications to shredders. With cryogenic grinding (grinding at very low temperatures—on the order of $-100°$ to $-200°$ centigrade —or $-148°$ to $-328°$ Fahrenheit), even more improvement seems possible. It has been reported that a conventional shredding process, processing cars cooled in liquid nitrogen (often used to cool objects to very low temperatures because its boiling point is $-195.8°C$), can remove 90–95 percent of the heterogeneous copper content of an automobile.[28] This would imply a final product with a copper content of 0.05–0.10 percent by weight,[29] depending on the amount of copper present in solution in the steel. In a telephone interview, an engineer who had experimented with cryogenic shredding[30] reported results similar to those given in the literature.

The additional costs incurred for equipment designed to remove further quantities of trace nonferrous impurities would be partially reimbursed by the recovery of the valuable impurities. Work by Huron Valley Corp.,[31] The Coreco Corp.,[32] Vanderbilt University,[33] and the U.S. Bureau of Mines[34] is aimed at more efficient recovery of the metallic

[27] See note 22.

[28] See "Fresh Frozen Scrap Produced by the INCH," *Industrial Research,* December 1970.

[29] In a publication which became available at the completion of the present study (N. A. Townsend, *Ferrous Scrap Processing,* distributed by National Technical Information Service, U.S. Department of Commerce, Bulletin PB-214 290, October 1972), it is reported that the firm of George and Sons, Liege, Belgium, has announced the development of a cryogenic fragmentizing process. Copper content of the product is reported to be about 0.08 percent.

[30] Telephone conversation with M. Levy, formerly employed by International Iron and Metal Company, Hamilton, Ontario, Canada, April 14, 1972.

[31] Telephone conversation with M. Wallace, Huron Valley Steel Corp., Bellville, Mich., October 23, 1972.

[32] Personal interview with D. Miller and M. Evans, College Research Corp., Milwaukee, Wis. at Institute of Scrap Iron and Steel Equipment Seminar, Chicago, May 1972.

[33] Vanderbilt University, Department of Physics and Astronomy, Annual Report, 1971, *Magnetic Separation of Non-Ferrous Metal* (Vanderbilt University, 1971).

[34] See R. L. Adams and S. E. Milanese, "An Economic Analysis of the Junk Auto with Emphasis on Processing Costs," *Proceedings of the Third Mineral Waste Utilization Symposium,* sponsored by the U.S. Bureau of Mines and IIT Research

TABLE 3-2. General Motors Analyses of Shredded Scrap: Amount of Constituent as Percent by Weight in Scrap

	Aluminum	Chromium	Copper	Lead	Molybdenum	Nickel	Tin	Zinc
Proler material	—	0.18	0.23	—	0.03	0.08	—	—
Luria material	—	0.24	0.21	—	0.03	0.22	—	—
First sampling S Allen system	0.03	0.11	0.12	0.10	—	0.17	0.05	0.03
Control test—6 cars S Allen system	—	0.14	0.12	—	—	0.17	—	—
S Allen system plus special processing by GM	—	0.11	0.07	0.01	—	0.19	0.04	0.01

Source: U.S. Congress, Senate, Committee on Public Works, *Resource Recovery Act of 1969 (Part 3)*, Hearings before the Subcommittee on Air and Water Pollution, Senate, on S. 2005, 91 Cong., 2 sess., 1970, pp. 1664, 1668.

values of the nonferrous fraction involved in the shredding operation.[35]

Finally, work is underway by the Ames, Iowa, AEC Laboratory, and by other researchers[36] on producing ultra-pure scrap. AEC workers find[37] that by melting conventional shredded scrap in an ultra-high vacuum (10^{-6} to 10^{-9} atmospheres), a steel product with 0.05 weight percent copper can be obtained.

Nevertheless, the fundamental question remains as to whether or not the value of higher quality steel scrap plus additional recovery of other metallic values is greater than the cost of the incremental inputs required for the additional processing.

Institute, Chicago, 1972; W. M. Mahan, "Foundry Iron Production from Automobile Scrap," *Proceedings of the Second Mineral Waste Utilization Symposium*, sponsored by the U.S. Bureau of Mines and IIT Research Institute, Chicago, 1970; P. C. Rosenthal, C. R. Loper, Jr., and R. W. Heine, "Technological Aspects of Utilizing Ferrous Urban Wastes," *Proceedings of the Third Mineral Waste Utilization Symposium*, sponsored by the U.S. Bureau of Mines and IIT Research Institute, Chicago, 1972; U.S. Department of the Interior, Bureau of Mines, *Recovery of the Non-Ferrous Metals from Auto Shredder Rejects by Air Classification*, by C. J. Chindgren, K. C. Dean, and LeRoy Peterson, Bureau of Mines Solid Waste Research Program, Technical Progress Report 31, 1971; Karl C. Dean, "Innovations in Recycling of Automotive Scrap," Paper presented at the 1972 Annual Convention of the Institute of Scrap Iron and Steel, Washington, D.C. (Reprinted in *Secondary Raw Materials*, vol. 10, no. 2, February 1972), January 1972.

[35] The Ford Motor Co. has even done research on the hydrolysis of the foam rubber (recovered from auto seats) produced by shredders to reduce its cost of disposal (L. R. Mahoney, S. A. Weiner, and F. C. Ferris, Ford Motor Co., Chemistry Department, *Hydrolysis of Polyurethane Foam*, Detroit, 1972; "Plastics Recycling Capability Expands," *Chemical and Engineering News*, May 22, 1972, p. 6).

[36] Makar *et al.* of the U.S. Bureau of Mines have worked on chemical means of removing copper from molten ferrous scrap, using sodium sulfate to slag off the copper. Their work (H. V. Makar, P. J. Gallagher, and R. E. Brown, "Removal of Copper from Molten Ferrous Scrap," *Proceedings of the Third Mineral Waste Utilization Symposium*, sponsored by the U.S. Bureau of Mines and IIT Research Institute, Chicago, 1972) indicates that copper levels can be reduced to 0.05 to 0.10 percent by weight by this technique, but no cost figures are available. If they started with a feed containing this level of copper, it is conceivable that they could produce an even lower copper concentration.

Cammarota, working with the U.S. Bureau of Mines (V. A. Cammarota, "Refining of Ferrous Metal Reclaimed from Municipal Incinerator Residues," *Proceedings of the Second Mineral Waste Utilization Symposium*, sponsored by the U.S. Bureau of Mines and IIT Research Institute, Chicago, 1970) has developed a method of processing the shredded ferrous fraction of municipal incinerator residues containing 0.2–0.5 percent copper and 0.1 to 0.4 percent tin, and reducing this, by leaching in aqueous ammonia solution, to 0.05 to 0.08 percent copper and 0.07 to 0.1 percent tin. He does not indicate projected costs for his method.

[37] See O. N. Carlson and F. A. Schmidt, *The Metallurgical Upgrading of Automotive Scrap Steel*, Report by the Ames Laboratory-USAEC, Iowa State University, 1972; F. A. Schmidt and O. N. Carlson, "The Removal of Copper, Tin and Chromium from Automotive Scrap Steel," Research Proposal of Department of Metallurgy, Iowa State University, 1970.

4

The Supply of
Deregistered Automobiles and Hulks

CALCULATING A DEREGISTRATION RATE COEFFICIENT

The supply of steel scrap derived from automobiles is partially determined by the rate at which automobiles are discarded. This rate can be estimated in a number of ways. Since this study is basically concerned with the next 10- to 15-year time span, the discard rate can be estimated by a single coefficient that describes the situation succinctly and that varies slowly with time.

There are currently about 7 million automobiles discarded annually in the United States in a population of about 210 million. Thus a disposal rate coefficient of 7/210, or 0.033 cars per person per year is generally applicable at present.[1] This "constant" will obviously vary with

---

[1] There is some indication, poorly documented but basically credible, that the 0.033 figure might vary to some extent from region to region. [See Tennessee Valley Authority, Office of Tributary Area Development, *From Field to Foundry* (Tennessee Valley Authority, 1972).] This is because, in very poor regions, the average car purchased is already quite old at the time of purchase and hence does not have the useful lifetime (to the last owner) of average cars in more affluent regions.

Other reasons for variations in the coefficient from region to region are also apparent. Some regions, for example, the Los Angeles area, have more cars per capita. New York City, on the other hand, may have considerably lower car ownership per capita than other areas. A thorough study of the coefficient and its variation in space and in time would require resources beyond the means of this study, and can reasonably be expected to yield information of marginal usefulness only.

Some background information which is of interest to the general problem of predicting automobile deregistrations is given by Adams; see Robert L. Adams, "An Economic Analysis of the Junk Automobile Problem," unpublished Ph.D. dissertation, University of Illinois, Department of Economics, Urbana, Illinois, 1972 (pp. 215–225). Attacking the deregistration problem, Adams reports sta-

37

time, since it will be related to the proportion of children in the total
population, the relative wealth of the population, the price of operating
automobiles, and a host of other factors. However, the 0.033 cars per
person per year disposal coefficient can reasonably be expected to vary
only slowly with time. It certainly seems plausible that over the next
5 years, for example, there will be very little change. Since the sub-
sequent analysis will show that the vast majority of the cars to be
deregistered, say 12 years from now, are those made from about 1 to 2
years ago to 4 to 5 years from now, a coefficient that remains relatively
time invariant for a 5-year span is sufficient for estimates of auto deregistrations for the next 10–12 years, which is the maximum time span
that will be considered in this study.[2] Thus this coefficient is sufficient
for the construction of a regional model of scrap supply. As the value
of the coefficient changes slowly over time, the coefficient in the model
may be changed accordingly.

The coefficient fails, however, to give other desirable information.
A long-range forecast, say 10–20 years, of the availability of deregistered
automobiles is of great interest to the steel industry, the scrap industry,
and the environmentalist. Appendix A of this chapter is devoted to this
problem, and includes a discussion of methods of forecasting the rate
of automobile deregistration and forecasts for each year until 1983.

---

tistical findings relating automobile registration by state to population, and finds
a high percentage of the variance accounted for (99.6 percent for 1967 data,
96.0 percent for 1968 data). He then reports the results of regressions of scrappage
estimates on auto registrations, and finds 92.2 percent of the variance accounted
for. Finally, he shows that auto registrations are negatively correlated with population density (studying only a few U.S. counties with exceptional population
densities) as well as population, that is, exceptionally crowded counties have
fewer automobiles than might be expected on the basis of population alone.
Taken as a whole, Adams' work supports the seemingly simplistic methodology
used in this study—to use a figure of 0.033 deregistrations per person per year
for a large region. While it undoubtedly is less than precise for a small and
atypical portion of the region, such as center city Philadelphia, it is probably a
good working estimate for the overall region within a 100-mile radius of Philadelphia.

[2] The purist may wish for a better estimate of the discard rate than given here.
It is not difficult to make one and incorporate it in the calculations. The procedure
is, briefly, to assume that the discard rate, referred to as r, is a function of time, t,
and can be expressed as a polynomial in t.

$$r = r(t) = a_0 + a_1 t + a_2 t^2 + a_3 t^3 + \ldots a_n t^n$$

The coefficient estimated in the text is merely a_0, and the other a_j's are assumed
to be zero.

Time series data are available on population data for the United States, and
time series data are available on deregistration data on automobiles in the United
States. Both these sets of time series data can be readily fit by polynomials of
low degree and merely dividing the two polynomials will yield an estimate of the
coefficients for the polynomial given above for $r(t)$.

The Problem of Aggregation

In any process analysis model of an industry, the problem of aggregation arises. There is an international scrap industry[3] that is composed of national scrap industries which are in turn composed of regional scrap processing industries (for example, those in the northeastern part of the United States).[4] These consist of metropolitan region scrap industries (such as Philadelphia and its environs) made up of individual scrap processors. The model maker must choose his level of aggregation carefully to satisfy some objective(s). His choice is constrained by data availability, the effort that can be expended, and the particular problems of concern to him.[5]

No general process analysis models of the scrap industry are available at any level of aggregation. There are two well-known process analysis models of the steel industry, those of Fabian[6] and Tsao and Day.[7]

---

[3] See N. J. G. Pound, "World Production and Use of Steel Scrap," *Economic Geography*, vol. 35, no. 3 (July 1959), pp. 249 ff.

[4] A good example of regional aggregation is provided by a series of reports by the U.S. Bureau of Mines on steel scrap in different regions of the United States (U.S. Department of the Interior, Bureau of Mines, *Iron and Steel Scrap in Arkansas, Kansas, Louisiana, Mississippi, Missouri, Oklahoma, and Texas*, by Frank B. Fulkerson and Harry F. Robertson, Bureau of Mines Information Circular 8289, 1966; U.S. Department of the Interior, Bureau of Mines, *Iron and Steel Scrap in California and Nevada*, by George C. Branner, Bureau of Mines Information Circular 7973, 1960; U.S. Department of the Interior, Bureau of Mines, *Iron and Steel Scrap in the Southeast*, by V. A. Danielson, James F. O'Neill, and H. William Ahrenholz, Bureau of Mines Information Circular 8329, 1967; U.S. Department of the Interior, Bureau of Mines, *Iron and Steel Scrap Survey in Illinois, Indiana, Iowa, Michigan, Minnesota, and Wisconsin*, by Walter Pajalich, Bureau of Mines Information Circular 8342, 1967). The series was never completed, and unfortunately one of the missing areas is the northeastern part of the United States.

[5] The current best-known example of models of a very high level of aggregation are those of Forrester [J. W. Forrester, *World Dynamics* (Wright-Allen Press, 1971)] and his associates at MIT, including Meadows [D. H. Meadows, D. L. Meadows, J. Randers, and W. W. Behrens III, *The Limits to Growth* (Universe Books, 1972)] and Randers (J. Randers, "The Dynamics of Solid Waste Generation," Preliminary draft report to The Club of Rome, Project on the Predicament of Mankind, by the Massachusetts Institute of Technology, Sloan School of Management Systems Dynamics Group, 1971). Randers' model is a nationally aggregated industrial dynamic model of the secondary copper industry.

[6] See Tibor Fabian, "Process Analysis of the U.S. Iron and Steel Industry," in *Studies in Process Analysis, Economy-Wide Production Capabilities*, A. A. Manne and H. M. Markowitz (eds.) (Wiley, 1961); Tibor Fabian, "A Linear Programming Model of Integrated Iron and Steel Production," *Management Science*, vol. 4, no. 4 (July 1958), pp. 415–449.

[7] C. E. Tsao, University of Massachusetts, Department of Economics, "A Process Analysis Model of the U.S. Steel Industry: Data Supplement," 1970 (mimeographed); C. S. Tsao and R. H. Day, "A Process Analysis Model of the U.S. Steel Industry," *Management Science*, vol. 17, no. 10 (1971), pp. 588 ff.

Both of these models are aggregated on the national scale. Fabian's goal was to aid in assessing national steelmaking capabilities[8] and Tsao and Day's study was made as part of a data base for a study of the steel industry's growth, Day's major interest. Hence, both of these studies naturally inclined toward a national aggregation.

The scrap industry, however, is of a regional nature mainly because of the high shipping costs (relative to the product value) incurred by scrap processors. Consider Philadelphia and its environs (within 100 miles). The sale price of No. 2 Bundles averaged from 1966 to 1972 about $21.50 per gross ton (see appendix A, chapter 7). The processing cost is about $3 per gross ton (see chapter 5). Raw material (auto hulks) costs are about $10 per gross ton plus transportation costs to the city, which are about $6 for the arbitrarily chosen 100-mile distance. Transportation cost to the steel mill is on the order of $0.03 per ton mile.[9] If the steel mill is located 100 miles away, the *total* transportation cost is $9, yielding the dealer a net loss of $0.50. This example makes it clear that the scrap processor simply cannot afford to ship either his raw material or his product very far, 100 to 200 miles being a representative limit. Thus it is natural to think in terms of aggregating all the scrap processors in a relatively large region surrounding some metropolis, rather than aggregating all the scrap processors in the United States.

The model developed in this study aggregates all scrap processors in the Philadelphia region and considers as its potential geographical supply and demand frontiers all the land area around Philadelphia in which it is profitable to buy or sell scrap automobiles. Stated in other words, all the scrap processors (and processes) within the Philadelphia area will be aggregated into one processor who will have available all the standard scrap processes at their current capacities with current or hypothetical environmental management factors and constraints included. This aggregated processor can buy and sell scrap from as far away as it is profitable to do so. That is, the mathematical structure of the model will simulate the behavior of the free market system in the Philadelphia region.

The model, however, is not limited to describing a region whose center of economic activity is Philadelphia. The approach is general. To apply this model to some other area, for instance, the region around Denver, it is only necessary to collect the relevant data for the Denver scrap industry and the population density distribution around Denver and use

    [8] Tibor Fabian, "Process Analysis of the U.S. Iron and Steel Industry," *Studies in Process Analysis*, p. 237.
    [9] See p. 44, Institute of Scrap Iron and Steel *Facts*, 31st ed. (Institute of Scrap Iron and Steel, Inc., 1971).

them in the model. Relevant data would include solid waste disposal charges in Denver, secondary materials prices, labor costs, and pollution regulations.

Population Distribution in the Philadelphia Region

At the beginning of this chapter it was estimated that about 0.033 automobiles per capita per year were deregistered. Using this coefficient, it is only necessary to have a knowledge of population density distribution in a region to estimate both the overall rate of deregistration and the location of the automobiles being deregistered. The population distribution of a geographic region surrounding a metropolitan area may be mathematically described in a number of ways. For the Philadelphia region, an analysis must concentrate on population within a specific section of the region and the average distance of that section from Philadelphia (in order to estimate transport costs). One scheme would be to determine the population in each census tract within some radius r (100–200 miles) from Philadelphia and then to consider the shipping distance for obsolete automobiles as the distance (Cartesian metric) from Philadelphia to the center of the census tract. A second and similar scheme might employ counties instead of census tracts. A third scheme might simply divide the section into square grids. The distance employed for the auto hulks being generated within each grid would be the distance from Philadelphia to the center of the grid. The simplest scheme, however, and that employed in the model, is to use a circular coordinate system, assume that variations of population density with respect to θ are relatively small compared with the variation of population density with respect to r, and treat the population sections as annuli at some distance from the center of the city.

The most important advantage of the circular coordinate approach is that it minimizes the number of variables. Let y_n represent the amount of material available from annulus n. The amount y_n will become part of the supply of Philadelphia scrap if the offering price in Philadelphia is greater than the price of the hulks at the source ($12) plus the shipping cost for annulus n. Even ten annuli give a fairly good description of the population density function, based on actual examination of the data. If the annuli are 10 miles wide, then a population density function covering a radius of up to 100 miles will cover a geographic area of 31,400 square miles. Describing the same supply function with grids 10 miles square would take 314 variables instead of 10. Thus, the use of a circular coordinate system offers a reduction by a factor of thirty in the number of variables required to describe the phenomenon.

It is clear that the price to be paid for the reduction in variables is a loss in accuracy, but (a) discussions of population distribution by both Isard[10] and Chorley and Haggett,[11] (b) an empirical study of the actual population density within a 100-mile radius of Philadelphia, and (c) the fact that shipping costs are *not* a function of θ but only of r, give assurance that the reduction in the number of variables by 90 percent is a sharp trade for the small loss in accuracy involved.

While the circular coordinate system has a powerful virtue, it also has a strong defect. It is inherently unsuited to modeling more than one center of population, that is, one center of scrap demand. In this study the model involves a central metropolitan region surrounded by country-side extending without practical limit. But this idealization is inadequate for regions with multiple demand centers. Should it be necessary to develop a regional model that incorporates more than one large scrap demand center, it would be advantageous to work in a rectangular coordinate system, and consider the standard census units, groups thereof, or counties as subregions.[12]

The circular coordinate approach was chosen for this study. The average population density within a 100-mile radius of Philadelphia can be well represented by the following equations:

$$\rho(r) = \begin{cases} 19200 \, e^{-0.284 \, r} & 0 \leq r \leq 9 \\ 1910 \, e^{-0.0274 \, r} & 9 \leq r \leq 100 \end{cases}$$

where ρ is population density per square mile and r is distance from center city Philadelphia in miles.[13]

---

[10] See W. Isard, *Location and Space Economy* (MIT Press, 1972), pp. 68–70.

[11] See R. J. Chorley and P. Haggett, *Models in Geography* [Methuen and Co., London (distributed in the United States by Barnes and Noble), 1967], pp. 343–344.

[12] Were such a scheme carried out for each major population region in the United States (a population produces scrap whether it is consumed or not), and the models then coupled, a national scrap model would result. Experiments on this model would demonstrate what levels of aggregation upward were valid. Moreover, this nationally aggregated model would be valuable not only for national policy studies, but for regional studies as well. For any point in the United States, this model would estimate the most economic disposition for obsolete steel products.

[13] The idea of using such an equation was developed by Colin Clark, and extensive verification is given by Berry *et al.* [See Colin Clark, "Urban Population Densities," *Journal of the Royal Statistical Society*, series A, vol. 114 (1951), pp. 490–496; B. J. L. Berry, J. W. Simmons, and R. J. Tennant, "Urban Population Densities: Structures and Change," *Geographical Review*, vol. 53 (1963), pp. 389–405.] The approach taken was to follow up on the suggestions of the regional scientists' work by making a short study of the population density within a 90-mile radius of Philadelphia, and then fit it with an appropriate empirical mathematical

function—along the lines of the relationships already prepared by mathematical geographic studies.

The procedure was as follows; the population density in persons per square mile was calculated for each county within 90 miles of Philadelphia. Next, the counties lying within annular rings of 15–20, 20–25, 25–30, 30–40, 40–50, 50–70, 70–90 miles, respectively, were found. Then the mean density within each annulus was found by averaging the included counties (omitting the New York City area). Utilizing this data it was found that

$$\rho = 1910 \ e^{-0.0274r} \qquad 15 \leq r \leq 90$$

with an r^2 (fraction variance removed) of 0.84 and a t test of 5.1, indicating a 99 + percent level of significance.

This good approximation of the empirical data was used to describe the population density in the area surrounding Philadelphia. It then remained to establish population density distribution within the central city. Data in the literature cited indicated

$$\rho = 66,000 \ e^{-0.40r} \qquad r < 12$$

These data were clearly outdated, since they were for 1940. The following procedure was adopted: let r_1 be the radius at the boundary between "center city" and "surrounding area." Then assume that the exponential decay pattern prevails but the constants ρ_0 and k differ depending on whether r is less than or greater than r_1. The population density then is

$$\rho(r) \begin{cases} \rho_0 e^{-kr} & r < r_1 \\ 1910 \ e^{-0.0274r} & r > r_1 \end{cases}$$

where $\rho(r)$ is the population density at radius r. Since the population density at the intersection of the two functions (that is, at r_1) must fit both functions, we have

$$\rho(r_1) = \rho_0 e^{-k_0 r_1}$$

$$\rho(r_1) = 1910.e^{-0.0274r_1}$$

Thus there is an interrelationship between r_1, ρ_0, and k_0. Using a careful estimate of the total population ($P = 5,460,000$) within a 40-mile radius of Philadelphia (that is, $r_2 = 40$), values of ρ_0 and k_0 were obtained for various values of r_1.

From the possible sets of values, r_1, ρ_0, k_0 equal to 9, 19200, 0.284, respectively, were chosen in the model. The average population density for Philadelphia County (1970 census) was 15,105 persons per square mile. Clearly this number is a lower limit for the value of ρ_0. Second, a value of k_0 in the neighborhood of 0.284 is plausibly close to what we might expect from the superannuated references available to us (Berry et al. and Clark). Regardless of what further research would reveal about the values of r_1, ρ_0, and k_0, repeated economic experiments run on the aggregated scrap processing model show that, at nearly any plausible factor costs for scrap, the automobile hulk scrap available from within 0–30 miles of Philadelphia has the highest priority in terms of consumption by scrap processors, because of its slightly lower transportation cost. Hence, the exact distribution of population within this radius is of minor consequence to the total supply curve being calculated.

TRANSPORTATION OF THE DEREGISTERED AUTO
TO THE DISMANTLER

The discussion above presents a methodology of predicting the rate of generation of deregistered automobiles and their location with respect to the central point of the region under consideration, Philadelphia. The first step in the automobile scrapping process (see figures 2-1 and 2-2) is transportation to a small scrap dealer. At the end of the useful life of an automobile, the (deregistered) automobile is (a) taken by the owner to a (usually) small scrap dealer, who gives the owner x_1 dollars for it, or (b) towed away by a (usually) small scrap dealer at the request of the owner, in which case the owner is usually paid nothing and it costs the scrap dealer x_2 dollars to tow it away, or (c) abandoned by the owner on a city street, or in a suburban or rural area. These latter cases cost the governmental unit involved some unknown and variable amount to detect and certify abandonment. Once this is done, it costs x_3 dollars for a scrap dealer to pick up the auto and tow it to his yard, or else the governmental unit itself does the towing.

A detailed examination of this portion of the scrapping process (an examination that would be a worthwhile piece of research) would reveal that x_1, x_2, and x_3 are all random variables of currently unknown distributions. This detailed information, which the systems analyst would like to have, is not yet available. However, interviews with numerous scrap dealers in the region around Philadelphia indicated that x_1, x_2, and x_3 were all about $10 on average (during 1972).[14] At first glance, this seems a happy coincidence. Some reflection, however, suggests that it is more than coincidence. Obsolete cars, whatever their source, are raw materials for the small scrap dealer. And the three possible sources discussed above are really competing with each other for the scrap dealer's purchasing dollar. Hence it is not surprising that the market tends to equilibrate, so that x_1, x_2, and x_3 are all approximately equal. This study, then, assumes that the same cost is incurred (this cost can be easily varied in the model, and in fact could be made into a random variable, with parameters varying with distance from some central point) for each and every automobile obtained by the small scrap dealer.[15] That is, this study will assume an infinite elasticity of supply

[14] The particular value used in the model is $10. It may, of course, easily be changed at the discretion of the user.

[15] It is of interest to examine briefly the case of an automobile that has a raw material price that is much greater than average because of locational disadvantage. For example, the car might be in a ravine, and it might cost the scrap dealer $20 to obtain it. Under what economic conditions will it be obtained? The evident answer is that it will be obtained by the scrap dealer when the price of scrap increases about $10 per ton and remains at about that level. But this is increasingly

of obsolete automobiles, for a given small geographic region, up to the limit of their availability—0.033 cars per person per year times the population of the region. When, for a given region, obsolete automobiles are being consumed as fast as they become available, the elasticity of supply is assumed to go to zero.

These assumptions about the supply of obsolete automobiles seem most realistic in exactly those regions of the country that are the major sources of automotive scrap, that is, regions of relatively high population density (100 persons per square mile and above) within 200–300 miles of large metropolitan centers such as Philadelphia. In regions of this type, obsolete automobiles are becoming available in any small subregion at a rate sufficient to justify the existence of a scrap dealer. This is not an unsupported assertion, for observations made during the course of the study consistently suggested that there are enough small scrap dealer–dismantling operations in the region around Philadelphia to ensure that there is almost always a dealer in the subregion under consideration who is able to either buy an obsolete automobile or obtain one for the cost of picking it up. In either case the cost is about the same as that incurred by other scrap dealers located in the entire general scrap market region under consideration. The model is most reliable, then, in those regions of the country which are the major sources of automotive scrap.

Summary

It may be helpful to summarize our conceptualization of the supply of deregistered automobiles. The geographical region around Philadelphia is seen as consisting of a series of annuli, each having some population density which is an empirically defined function of the radial distance of that annulus from Philadelphia.

The annuli consist of an undefined number of small regions. Each region is sufficiently large (in terms of automobiles deregistered) to make it profitable for one scrap dealer to be in business dismantling deregistered automobiles. Any specific scrap dealer, in a specific region, in any of the annuli, can buy as many deregistered automobiles as he

---

unlikely to happen, for it is demonstrated herein that the short-term elasticity of supply of steel scrap is quite high, probably at least five, and growing higher. This high elasticity arises from the fact that hulk transportation costs are so low. Thus, ironically, it is probably already cheaper for an "average" (that is, a $10) obsolete automobile to be shipped from, say Binghamton, N Y., to a scrap dealer in Philadelphia (150 miles) than it is for a locationally disadvantaged (that is, a $20) obsolete automobile to be shipped from the outskirts of Philadelphia to a scrap dealer in Philadelphia.

likes—for a constant price—up to the point at which he is buying all the automobiles which the population in that region deregisters (which is defined as the population of the region times the deregistration rate coefficient, valued at 0.033 cars per person per year). That is, as long as he is buying at a rate less than that at which cars are being deregistered, the elasticity of supply of cars is infinite. When he attempts to buy cars at a rate greater than that at which they are being deregistered, the elasticity of supply becomes zero.

After the cars are dismantled, a process that will be described in chapter 5, they are shipped to the hulk processor. This shipping step will be discussed in chapter 6 along with hulk processing.

APPENDIX A
Forecast of Deregistered Auto Availability

The data necessary for the prediction of deregistered automobile availability are data on registration of cars by year of production. These data are not readily available to the researcher for any geographic region less than the nation as a whole.[16]

The Motor Vehicle Manufacturers Association annually publishes nationally aggregated data on automobile production, imports, exports, and the number of deregistrations. Deregistrations are the closest thing to what the scrap supply analyst might term "availability" data and are used by the Motor Vehicle Manufacturers Association and others to estimate the same.

Using the Motor Vehicle Manufacturers Association data on registration[17] and purchase data (production plus imports minus exports), the average probability that an auto will survive (that is, not be deregistered) the nth year after its manufacture can be calculated. From these data

---

[16] These data are available, for a fee, from R. L. Poke and Co., Inc. of Detroit, Mich., which maintains extensive files on automobile registration, by political district (county), and will sell such data.

[17] Motor Vehicle Manufacturers Association of the U.S., Inc., *1971 Automobile Facts and Figures* (Motor Vehicle Manufacturers Association of the U.S., Inc., 1971).

it is a simple matter to calculate the probability that a car will be taken out of registration in year n (after manufacture). These data are shown in table 4-1 for autos produced from 1946 to 1968.[18] Moreover, the average probability survival data for cars made from 1946 to 1968 are compared with similar data from 1941, 1954, 1955, and 1956 (this

---

[18] Values for the first year are estimated, since no data are available, while for the second year the data are questionable owing to registration ambiguities (see table 4-1). Therefore, these data are obtained by interpolation.

Data for years past 15 are not available, but are readily calculated (extrapolated) from the knowledge that, after a period of 10–11 years, the removal of cars from registration can be described by a simple exponential decay model. That is (see figure 4-1), since

$$\ln p = k_1 - k_2 t$$
then
$$p = e^{k_1 - k_2 t} = k_3 e^{-k_2 t}$$

There is, unfortunately, no way of knowing how far such an extrapolation is reliable. The data seem to indicate that automobile lifetimes are surprisingly constant, in view of the oft-expressed notion that automobiles "don't last like they used to." Nonetheless, the values calculated should be taken as guideline approximations, rather than fundamental constants.

TABLE 4-1. Statistical Data on Automobile Survival[a]

Year n	Probability that a car will survive its nth year	Probability that a car will be taken out of registration in year n
1	0.984[b]	0.016[b]
2	0.968[b]	0.016[b]
3	0.951	0.017
4	0.932	0.019
5	0.905	0.027
6	0.876	0.029
7	0.811	0.065
8	0.729	0.082
9	0.607	0.122
10	0.483	0.124
11	0.362	0.121
12	0.278	0.084
13	0.209	0.069
14	0.156	0.053
15	0.113	0.043
16	0.087[b]	0.026[b]
17	0.0655[b]	0.0215[b]
18	0.0491[b]	0.0164[b]
19	0.0367[b]	0.0124[b]
20	0.0272[b]	0.0095[b]

Source: Motor Vehicle Manufacturers Association of the U.S., Inc., 1972 Automobile Facts and Figures (Detroit, Michigan: Motor Vehicle Manufacturers Association of the U.S., 1972).
[a] All data averages for production from 1945 to 1968.
[b] Estimates.

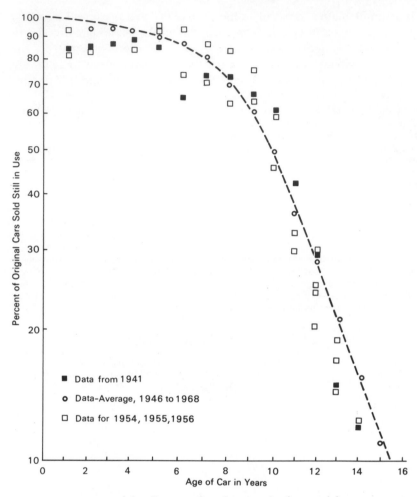

FIGURE 4-1.   Percent of total car production surviving.

latter obtained from Brown[19]) in figure 4-1, in which the log of the
percentage of cars still in use in a given year is plotted as a function of
the age of car in years.[20] Data for 1941 are for cars produced in 1927
in their fifteenth year of service, cars produced in 1928 in their four-

---

[19] See R. G. Brown, *Smoothing, Forecasting and Prediction of Discrete Time
Series* (Prentice-Hall, 1963), p. 260.

[20] The plot is on a semilog basis because this brings out a key feature of the
data. Following an initial period of time during which the probability that a car
is deregistered during a given year varies, this probability finally becomes constant,
as is indicated by the *straight line section of the curve* on the semilog plot after
about 9–10 years.

teenth year of service, and so forth. As a social phenomenon, reflecting the behavior of U.S. citizens from 1927 to 1968, the data in figure 4-1 exhibit a surprising uniformity of pattern. Indeed, the uniformity is sufficient to suggest that the deregistration probability pattern of automobiles discussed above can serve as a basis for the construction of a simple, credible, and hopefully reliable method of predicting automobile deregistrations.

Domestic automobile purchases in year t are the sum of domestic production plus imports minus exports. Using these data, a time series of purchases can be constructed. This time series, starting with 1950 (a date chosen to try to minimize the effect of discontinuities in purchasing patterns arising from World War II) can be used to predict domestic auto purchases for the future. Finally, deregistration rates may be estimated from the predicted values for auto purchases and the probabilities of deregistration already calculated.

The method used to mathematically organize auto purchasing data was triple exponential smoothing of the time series.[21] This method not only yields a predicted set of future values of the time series being studied, but also yields "reasonable" upper and lower limit values for the time series in question. The history of auto purchases since 1950 and the predicted future values with their expected errors, as calculated by the triple exponential smoothing technique, are shown in table 4-2. Deregistration rates may be predicted from the predicted values for auto purchases (table 4-2) and the probabilities of deregistration already calculated. There are two errors associated with the prediction of deregistrations: one from the variations in the probabilities of deregistration, assumed to be negligible in the absence of other information, and one from the errors in the predicted values of the purchases. One set of the deregistration predictions (table 4-3) given is based on the predicted value of purchases, one set of predictions is based on the low values predicted for purchases, and one set of predictions is based on the high values predicted for purchases (see table 4-2). All these predictions are given in table 4-3 for each year until 1983. The errors in prediction are included in the table for the years 1950–1969. In the early part of this time span, the errors in deregistration prediction are understandably large since the predicted values are highly dependent upon previous purchase patterns (because of the 10-year lag between purchases and deregistration), which were very abnormal during and immediately after World War II. Starting with 1958, reflecting purchase

---

[21] See R. G. Brown, *Smoothing, Forecasting,* chapters 8, 11, 12, 16; IBM Corp., *System/360 Scientific Subroutine Package (360A-CM-03X) Programmer's Manual (Publication No. H20-0205-0)* (IBM Corp., 1966), pp. 40, 41. The technique of triple exponential smoothing is explained fully in Brown's book.

TABLE 4-2.   Past and Predicted U.S. Automobile Purchases in Millions

Year	Actual purchases	Predicted purchases	Predicted low purchases	Predicted high purchases
1950	6.534	5.390	—	—
1951	5.193	5.624	—	—
1952	4.163	5.642	—	—
1953	5.946	5.513	—	—
1954	5.375	5.687	—	—
1955	7.723	5.769	—	—
1956	5.718	6.219	—	—
1957	6.115	6.322	—	—
1958	4.359	6.486	—	—
1959	5.791	6.370	—	—
1960	6.974	6.496	—	—
1961	5.853	6.800	—	—
1962	7.255	6.905	—	—
1963	7.970	7.223	—	—
1964	8.095	7.624	—	—
1965	9.660	8.007	—	—
1966	9.028	8.596	—	—
1967	8.337	9.027	—	—
1968	9.656	9.307	—	—
1969	9.528	9.762	—	—
1970	8.397	10.157	—	—
1971	10.247	10.323	—	—
1972	—	10.831	9.423	12.239
1973	—	11.301	9.746	12.856
1974	—	11.789	10.126	13.453
1975	—	12.297	10.542	14.052
1976	—	12.824	10.989	14.658
1977	—	13.369	11.462	15.276
1978	—	13.934	11.959	15.908
1979	—	14.517	12.480	16.554
1980	—	15.119	13.022	17.217
1981	—	15.740	13.586	17.895
1982	—	16.381	14.171	18.590
1983	—	17.040	14.777	19.304

patterns about 10 years earlier, predictions are within about 10 percent or less of the actual values.[22]

The predictions of auto deregistrations in table 4-3 are based on a (relatively) crude analysis of auto purchase and a (relatively) sophisticated analysis of the deregistration process. Other data are available from the U.S. Department of Transportation[23] and are based on a (rela-

[22] The actual equation for automobile purchases developed by the triple exponential smoothing technique is:

$$P(t) = 10,380,530. + 441206. (t\text{-}1972) + 18965. (t\text{-}1972)^2$$

[23] See U.S. Congress, Senate Committee on Public Works, *Resource Recovery Act of 1969 (Part 3)*, Hearings before the Subcommittee on Air and Water Pollution, Senate, on S. 2005, 91 Cong., 2 sess., 1970, pp. 1679, 1680.

TABLE 4-3.   Past and Predicted Deregistrations in the U.S. in Millions

Year	Actual deregistration	Predicted deregistration	Predicted low deregistration	Predicted high deregistration	Percent error
1950	2.598	2.543	—	—	− 2.1
1951	3.122	2.326	—	—	−25.5
1952	3.163	2.064	—	—	−34.7
1953	3.466	1.859	—	—	−46.4
1954	3.840	1.914	—	—	−50.2
1955	3.773	2.124	—	—	−43.7
1956	4.327	2.523	—	—	−41.7
1957	3.703	3.003	—	—	−18.9
1958	3.639	3.510	—	—	− 3.5
1959	4.413	3.928	—	—	−10.9
1960	4.200	4.325	—	—	3.0
1961	4.401	4.606	—	—	4.7
1962	4.773	4.896	—	—	2.6
1963	5.174	5.129	—	—	− 0.9
1964	6.064	5.460	—	—	−10.0
1965	6.163	5.593	—	—	− 9.2
1966	6.056	5.757	—	—	− 4.9
1967	6.433	5.829	—	—	− 9.4
1968	6.266	5.973	—	—	− 4.7
1969	5.894	6.180	—	—	4.8
1970	—	6.467	—	—	—
1971	—	6.739	—	—	—
1972	—	7.105	—	—	—
1973	—	7.498	7.476	7.521	—
1974	—	7.884	7.837	7.932	—
1975	—	8.224	8.149	8.300	—
1976	—	8.523	8.415	8.631	—
1977	—	8.781	8.628	8.934	—
1978	—	9.068	8.864	9.273	—
1979	—	9.360	9.502	9.669	—
1980	—	9.712	9.268	10.115	—
1981	—	10.096	9.452	10.739	—
1982	—	10.569	9.709	11.429	—
1983	—	11.043	9.961	12.126	—

tively) sophisticated analysis of auto purchases. These results are briefly summarized here (see table 4-4) and used with the method developed in this study for predicting deregistration. This is done for purposes of completeness and because their usage points up an important fact. Even though the Department of Transportation's predictions of purchases of automobiles are far less than those calculated herein, the calculated obsolete auto availability is nearly the same (see table 4-3). This arises from the important fact that the great bulk of scrap available 10 years from time t is produced within the range of $t − 3$ to $t + 3$ years. Hence, while it may be difficult to predict automobile purchases 10 years in advance, it is relatively easy to predict them 3 or 4 years in advance, and therefore scrap availability may be predicted, for 10 years in advance, far more accurately than automobile purchases.

TABLE 4-4.   Data on Automobile Purchases and Deregistrations[a]

Year	Auto purchases in millions (estimated)	Auto deregistration in millions (estimated) U.S. Dept. of Transportation	U.S. Dept. of Transportation purchase estimates—Our method of deregistration calculation	Our purcha. estimates—Our method of deregistration calculation
1969	9.7	6.8	6.18	6.18
1970	10.0	7.5	6.47	6.47
1971	10.0	7.6	6.74	6.74
1972	10.1	7.8	7.10	7.10
1973	10.2	8.0	7.49	7.50
1974	10.4	8.2	7.85	7.88
1975	10.7	8.6	8.17	8.22
1976	10.9	8.7	8.44	8.52
1977	11.2	8.9	8.66	8.78
1978	11.3	9.1	8.90	9.07
1979	11.6	9.4	9.10	9.36
1980	11.8	9.6	9.33	9.71
1981	12.0	9.8	9.54	10.10
1982	12.3	10.2	9.80	10.57
1983	12.4	10.3	10.02	11.04

[a] Data from U.S. Department of Transportation, Federal Highway Administration, Bureau of Public Roads.

5

The Dismantling Model

After transportation to a scrap dealer, the next step in the gradual transformation of a deregistered automobile into processed scrap is dismantling. In the automobile sector of the scrap business, there are: (a) dealers who dismantle (and usually salvage to some extent), (b) dealers who dismantle and then further process (such as shear or bale), and (c) dealers who essentially only process. The first and third categories are dominant (see figures 2-1 and 2-2). That is, broadly speaking, the scrap industry can be considered as having two separate sectors— dealers who dismantle and dealers who process.

Thus, the dismantling sector of the automobile scrapping industry can be conceptually separated from the processing sector.[1] This fact immediately suggests the approach taken here to modeling the scrap industry as a whole: that is, to make two submodels, the first dealing with dismantling, the second dealing with processing (in the more conventional sense of the term).

An automobile is a complex piece of equipment. Depending on the level of aggregation considered, it can be thought of as having 1,000 parts (the left front interior door handle, the left rear interior door handle, etc.); 100 parts; or on the other extreme, 2 parts (the metallic part and the nonmetallic part). The level of aggregation that a study considers is not, however, a matter of arbitrary choice. It must reflect the economic effects of parts removal—the value of the remainder of the automobile

---

[1] Viewed abstractly, the dismantling operations (of a firm that both salvages and dismantles) may be considered separately from the salvaging operations of the same firm. Salvaging refers to selling a part from a used car as a replacement part.

and the cost of taking out the part. Keeping this end in mind, the classification of auto parts offered by Dean and Sterner[2] provides an excellent starting point for defining what parts ought to be specifically considered. In their study of this problem, they considered an automobile as consisting of thirty-six parts. They dismantled fifteen automobiles manufactured between 1954 and 1965 and measured: (a) the average time required for the removal of each of the parts; (b) the average time required for the disassembly of each part for the recovery of the salable nonferrous metals; and (c) the amount of nonferrous metals (of at least some type) in each of the parts, hence their potential sale value. Their results are shown in table 5-2 in appendix A[3] of this chapter.

Consider an automobile as consisting of n parts. For any specific part m, the following actions are possible (see figure 5-1):

1. Remove part m
2. If removed, disassemble or do not disassemble
3. If removed but not disassembled, sell as is or do not sell as is
4. If removed but not sold as is, and not disassembled, dispose of as solid waste

The algorithm can be expressed verbally for part m:

1. If the sale price of the part exceeds the cost of removal, or if the sale prices of the metals of which the part is composed exceed the cost of removal and disassembly, remove the part.
2. If removed, and if the sale price of the part (there is a market for a number of parts—e.g., "copper-bearing material" includes the disassembled electric motors and generators, and sells for about 1¼ cents per pound) is greater than or equal to the sale prices of the metal components minus the cost of disassembly, sell the part without disassembling. Otherwise, disassemble the part and sell its metal components.
3. If removed (because its removal is demanded by the hulk processor) and not salable (for example, tires), dispose of as solid waste.[4]

---

[2] See U.S. Department of the Interior, Bureau of Mines, *Dismantling a Typical Junk Automobile to Produce Quality Scrap*, Bureau of Mines Report of Investigations 7350, 1969.

[3] See Joseph W. Sterner, *Weights and Types of Metals and Nonmetals in 1957 Ford 4-Door, Hardtop Sedan with Automatic Transmission*, Memo to K. C. Dean, Salt Lake City Metallurgy Research Center, Bureau of Mines, U.S. Department of the Interior, February 17, 1967; and U.S. Department of the Interior, Bureau of Mines, *Dismantling a Typical Junk Automobile.*

[4] Shredders cannot usually cope with tires because of their physical properties. Thus, they must be removed before shredding.

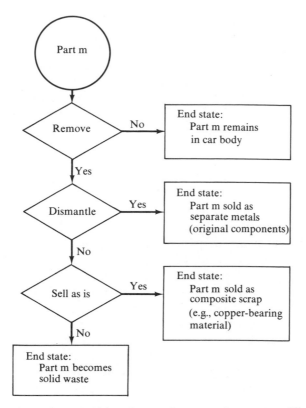

FIGURE 5-1.   Decision diagram for part *m* in an automobile.

Consider the imposition of a further condition: namely that the concentration of some particular nonferrous metal in the hulk is constrained to be less than or equal to a particular value. Mathematically this extension to the algorithm is also straightforward. After calculating the relevant costs of removal and dismantling, and calculating the profit from selling as is or selling the dismantled parts, continue to remove parts containing the tramp metal, in order of decreasing profit (even if negative), until the constraint is satisfied.

There are a number of contaminants (about five) which might reasonably be constrained, and it is commonplace for some parts to contain a number of nonferrous contaminants (see appendix A of this chapter, table 5-4). An analysis of bumpers from one model car, for example, indicates a weight of 79.5 pounds and the presence of 0.0016 pounds aluminum, 0.0075 pounds copper, 0.175 pounds chromium, 0.038 pounds manganese, 0.0239 pounds molybdenum, and 2.0 pounds of nickel.[5] All of these nonferrous elements are of concern to the steel-maker. Moreover, as was discussed in chapter 3, the steelmaker might like to constrain the sum of the concentrations of these five nonferrous elements and sometimes both the concentrations of the individual elements and the sum of the concentrations of the elements.

This multiple constraint problem defies solution by the simple algorithm described above.[6] A more general method is necessary for attacking the problem of optimum dismantling. Even if the method used did not determine the globally optimum activity levels, it would be of value if it offered an approximation. Moreover, it would be highly desirable if the method proposed allowed the ready determination of variations in optimal activity levels with changes in the prices of labor, raw materials (car bodies), products, and by-product disposal. As a result, the problem described above was formulated as a mixed integer linear programming problem. The equations formally describing the mathematical model are included as appendix B of this chapter.

A new technological development, the engine puller, may replace part of the hand dismantling process. It is a tractor-mounted, hydraulically powered device used to pull out the engine of an automobile and those items integrally attached to the engine. These items include the flywheel housing, starter-solenoid set, generator, coil, voltage regulator, thermostat, fuel pump, carburetor, distributor, and engine wiring. All other parts which can be removed from the car must be removed manually. The engine pulling process is mentioned by Adams[7] as one which could possibly enjoy widespread use in the future. Therefore, a second automobile dismantling model was made using an engine puller. Mathematically it is exactly equivalent to the hand dismantling process, with only one exception: the removal of the engine and its integrally associated parts are aggregated together as one variable.[8] Experiments with this second dismantling model have been limited to those required to assure the elimination of all infeasibilities. The few experiments run seemed to

[5] This analysis is from the Bureau of Mines for a 1957 Ford (Joseph W. Sterner, *Weights and Types of Metals*). Interviews with steel company representatives, however, indicate that bumper composition varies considerably.

[6] See R. Dorfman, P. A. Samuelson, and R. M. Solow, *Linear Programming and Economic Analysis* (McGraw-Hill, 1958).

[7] See R. L. Adams, "An Economic Analysis of the Junk Automobile Problem," unpublished Ph.D. dissertation, Department of Economics, University of Illinois, 1972.

[8] In the construction of the dismantling models, we have used the same rows for both methods of dismantling, thereby eliminating much redundancy. The models may be separated by the user should he so desire. If this is not done, the user must ensure that there is no coupling between the two independent models. In IBM's linear programming packages (MPS or MPSX) this is readily accomplished by "flagging" the columns (activities) not being used (in this case, the entire submodel).

indicate that, at current materials prices, the engine puller mode of operation is slightly less profitable (about $1 per car less) than hand dismantling of all parts.

The dismantling models described above are in the form of mixed integer linear programming problems. The parts and secondary materials prices are in the objective function, and equations between the variables (activities) constrain the solution to the physically feasible. The problem is linear because, for every activity, multiplying the level of that activity by k will result in multiplying the cost (or profit) associated with the activity by k.

The models consider an automobile as consisting of forty parts. The removal (or not) of each part is an activity, its sale as is (or not) is an activity, its disassembly (or not) is an activity, and its disposition as solid waste (or not) is an activity. Moreover, numerous other variables are also included; for example, the amount of each type of metal produced to be sold (noninteger variables) and the amounts of the various metals remaining in the hulk after dismantling (noninteger variables). Material balance and number balance equations are included in the model and relate all these activities.

VERIFICATION

If correct, the model should, given a currently typical set of labor, materials prices, and residuals discard costs, predict the production of automobile hulks with about the same composition as No. 2 Bundles, since there is no removal of tramp elements in the transformation of a stripped automobile hulk in a baling operation. Accordingly, a computer run was made with the dismantling model with no quality constraints, and the composition data shown in table 5-1 were obtained for the five tramp elements of greatest interest.

These results help to verify the model. Other evidence verifying the reliability of the calculations was also obtained. For example, at current secondary metals prices, the calculations indicate that the nonferrous elements *not* removed are present in the dismantled hulk in the following quantities: zinc die castings, 48.6 pounds; aluminum, 11.8 pounds; copper, 11.2 pounds; chromium, 9.0 pounds. As percentages of the total nonferrous material present, these amount to about 60 percent for zinc, 15 percent for aluminum, 14 percent for copper, and 11 percent chromium. These figures correspond with data reported by Roos[9] for

---

[9] R. V. Roos, "Magnetic Separation of Nonferrous Metal," in Annual Report, Department of Physics and Astronomy, Vanderbilt University, Nashville, Tenn., 1971.

TABLE 5-1. Amount of Five Nonferrous Metallic Elements in a
Dismantled Automobile

Metal	Calculated percent by weight remaining in hulk	Actual percent by weight reported in No. 2 Bundles[a]
Copper	0.49	0.48
Chromium[b]	0.39	0.06
Molybdenum	0.03	0.03
Nickel	0.06	0.09
Tin	0.05	0.06
Total	1.02	0.72

[a] These results are from W. L. Swager, *The Measurement and Improvement of Scrap Quality*, Battelle Memorial Institute, Columbus, Ohio, Nov. 30, 1960; and C. C. Custer, "The Quality Aspects of a Cold Metal Practice vs. a Hot Metal Practice," Paper presented at the Forty-Seventh National Open Hearth and Basic Oxygen Steel Conference, AIME, April 13, 1964. Cited by W. J. Regan *et al.*, *Final Report on Identification of Opportunities for Increased Recycling of Ferrous Solid Waste*, Report by the Battelle Memorial Institute to the Scrap Metal Research and Education Foundation of the Institute of Scrap Iron and Steel, Inc. (Washington, D.C.: Institute of Scrap Iron and Steel, Inc., 1972).
[b] The error in chromium is partially explained by the fact that the chromium contents from melts is apt to be less than the amount of chromium in the feed, owing to losses in the slag. This does not completely eliminate the problem, however. Careful examination of the analytical data reveals further difficulties. Table 3-1 in this study indicates chromium content of shredded scrap to be 0.16 percent, with chromium content of No. 2 Bundles at 0.06 percent (Custer's value for chromium). But the hulks for No. 2 Bundle production and shredded scrap production are dismantled, as far as we have been able to ascertain, the same way. The data contain some anomalies that are not easily explained.

nonferrous input to shredders as 60 percent zinc die cast, 23 percent aluminum, 10 percent copper, and 7 percent stainless steel. This is taken as further evidence that the model is accurately describing the hand dismantling process.[10]

[10] There is a problem in the comparison of these two sets of figures. The poundages are calculated from a composite average of the composition and removal time figures for fifteen cars as reported by the Bureau of Mines study (*Dismantling a Typical Junk Automobile*), the cars examined ranging from a 1954 to a 1965 model. The data from Roos are composite data for cars currently (1971–1972) entering a shredder in Tennessee. It must be assumed that, to a first approximation, the automobiles entering the shredder in Tennessee are similar in composition to those so carefully examined by the Bureau of Mines. This is a reasonable assumption, since auto lifetime data strongly support the notion that autos being deregistered in 1971–1972 are models of the time period 1958 to 1965.

APPENDIX A

Relevant Data for Automobile Dismantling Model

TABLE 5-2, Part 1. Bureau of Mines Auto Dismantling Data

Part	Weight (pounds)	Removal time (minutes) Part	Non-ferrous metals	Cu as Cu	Copper as yellow brass	Copper from yellow brass	Alum	Zinc	Cast iron	Light iron	Heavy iron
Battery, cable and clamps	36.5	1.6	0.3	0.8	0.0	0.0	0.0	0.0	0.0	0.0	0.0
Radiator	14.5	5.4	1.8	13.0	0.0	0.0	0.0	0.0	0.0	0.0	0.0
Engine	454.5	4.8	44.2	0.0	0.0	0.0	12.5	0.0	374.0	12.0	56.0
Differential	153.5	8.1	0.0	0.0	0.3	0.2	0.0	0.0	51.2	17.3	84.7
Flywheel housing	9.4	2.7	0.6	0.0	0.0	0.0	8.7	0.0	0.0	0.0	0.7
Starter and solenoid	15.5	2.0	10.3	2.8	0.0	0.0	1.0	0.0	0.0	0.2	11.5
Generator	12.0	1.1	7.1	2.6	0.0	0.0	1.5	0.0	0.0	2.9	4.9
Coil	2.0	0.7	2.4	0.5	0.0	0.0	0.0	0.0	0.0	1.1	0.0
Voltage regulator	1.1	0.4	0.5	0.2	0.7	0.5	0.0	0.0	0.0	0.9	0.0
Thermostat	0.7	0.9	0.2	0.0	0.3	0.2	0.0	0.0	0.0	0.5	0.0
Fuel pump	3.5	3.0	5.9	0.0	0.3	0.2	0.8	2.0	0.0	0.4	0.0
Carburetor	6.5	0.4	4.1	0.0	0.0	0.0	1.1	3.8	1.5	0.3	0.0
Distributor	4.0	1.0	2.6	0.4	0.0	0.0	0.3	0.3	2.7	0.0	0.5
Engine wiring	0.5	1.5	0.2	0.8	0.0	0.0	0.0	0.0	0.0	0.0	0.0
Electric motors	8.9	4.7	5.0	2.4	0.0	0.0	1.5	1.8	0.0	2.6	2.1
Heater core	8.2	4.4	2.4	0.8	0.0	0.0	0.0	0.0	0.0	0.0	0.0
Dashboard wiring	2.3	6.5	0.3	2.4	0.0	0.0	0.0	0.0	0.0	0.3	0.0
Instruments	3.9	0.8	1.7	0.0	0.7	0.5	0.0	1.8	0.0	0.8	0.0
Radio	4.6	0.9	8.7	0.3	0.0	0.0	0.0	2.0	0.0	1.8	0.0

TABLE 5-2, Part 2. Bureau of Mines Auto Dismantling Data

Part	Weight (pounds)	Removal time (minutes)		Weight of metal in the part (pounds)								
		Part	Non-ferrous metals	Cu as Cu	Copper as yellow brass	Copper from yellow brass	Alum	Zinc	Cast iron	Light iron	Heavy iron
Interior trim	21.1	9.7	16.2	0.0	0.0	0.0	1.5	16.2	0.0	3.4	0.0
Body wiring	7.2	16.6	0.3	4.0	0.0	0.0	0.0	0.0	0.0	0.6	0.0
Mirrors, light covers	12.0	0.4	1.4	0.0	0.0	0.0	0.0	1.8	0.0	0.3	0.0
Interior handles	3.6	3.1	7.3	0.0	0.0	0.0	0.0	3.4	0.0	0.2	0.0
Exterior handles	4.2	4.3	4.6	0.0	0.0	0.0	0.0	4.2	0.0	0.0	0.0
Horn and relay	3.3	1.2	24.5	0.2	0.0	0.0	0.0	2.1	0.0	1.1	0.0
Tubing	2.1	5.3	1.1	0.4	0.0	0.0	0.0	0.0	0.0	1.7	0.0
Exterior trim and grill	15.5	7.2	17.1	0.0	0.0	0.0	6.4	8.1	0.0	0.8	0.2
Window frames	11.4	6.9	11.2	0.0	0.0	0.0	0.0	6.7	0.0	4.7	0.0
Transmission	153.8	9.2	14.5	0.0	0.3	0.2	15.3	0.0	3.6	19.5	115.1
Brake drums and cylinders	79.4	7.1	4.1	0.0	0.3	0.2	0.0	0.0	73.2	2.3	3.6
Bumpers and trim	79.5	0.0	0.0	0.0	0.0	0.0	0.0	0.0	0.0	79.5	0.0
Body trim and decoration	4.8	0.0	0.0	0.0	0.0	0.0	0.0	0.0	0.0	4.8	0.0
Steering gear box	8.0	0.0	0.0	0.0	0.0	0.0	0.0	0.0	5.2	1.3	1.5
Wheel covers and wheels	78.7	4.2	0.0	0.0	0.0	0.0	0.0	0.0	0.0	9.9	68.8
Light iron	1136.8	0.0	0.0	0.0	0.0	0.0	0.0	0.0	0.0	1136.8	0.0
Heavy iron	874.3	0.0	0.0	0.0	0.0	0.0	0.0	0.0	0.0	0.0	874.3
Total of each metal	3179.3	124.1	200.6	29.2	2.9	2.0	50.6	54.2	511.4	1309.5	1222.4

Source: U.S. Department of the Interior, Bureau of Mines, *Dismantling a Typical Junk Automobile to Produce Quality Scrap,* Bureau of Mines Report of Investigations 7350. (Washington, D.C.: Government Printing Office, 1969).

TABLE 5-3.   Analysis of Main Components in 1957 Ford, 4-Door, Hardtop Sedan

Part or type metal	Analysis (%)						
	C	S	Al	Cu	Si	Zn	Pb
Pistons	—	—	80.4	3.1	10.0	0.9	—
Transmission	—	—	83.0	3.62	10.4	0.8	—
Heater and core	—	—	—	58.95	—	12.1	21.5
Radiator	—	—	—	72.3	—	4.0	17.5
Grill	—	—	—	0.2	0.14	—	0.01
Trim	—	—	0.03	0.35	0.40	—	—
Zinc die cast	—	—	3.94	0.45	0.04	—	—
Light steel	1.5	< 0.01	0.09	0.05[a]	1.85	—	0.002
Heavy steel[a]	0.31	< 0.01	< 0.01	0.015[a]	0.06	—	< 0.001
Forged steel[a]	1.05	0.01	0.28	0.21[a]	0.25	—	—
Cast iron[a]	3.4	0.09	0.02	0.12[a]	2.06	—	0.37
Bumper	—	—	0.02	0.11	0.40	—	—

	Sn	Fe	Cr	Ni	Mn	Mg
Pistons	—	2.33	—	0.4	0.1	1.56
Transmission	—	1.0	—	0.1	0.1	0.5
Heater and core	3.74	3.4	—	—	—	—
Radiator	4.02	2.1	—	—	—	—
Grill	—	96.5	0.20	0.1	0.6	—
Trim	—	80.0	16.5	0.29	0.3	—
Zinc die cast	—	93.7	—	0.85	—	—
Light steel	0.006	95.0	0.1	0.063	0.3	—
Heavy steel[a]	0.007	98.0	0.03	0.044	0.4	—
Forged steel[a]	—	96.0	0.73	0.20	0.8	—
Cast iron[a]	0.018	92.7	0.32	0.12	0.8	—
Bumper	—	93.7	0.22	2.27	0.5	—

	SiO_2	CaO	Na_2O	MgO	Al_2O_3	B_2O_3
Glass	70.8	8.4	12.7	3.7	0.8	N.D.[b]

Source: Joseph W. Sterner, *Weights and Types of Metals and Nonmetals in 1957 Ford 4-Door, Hardtop Sedan with Automatic Transmission.* Memo to K. C. Dean, Salt Lake City Metallurgy Research Center, Bureau of Mines, U.S. Department of the Interior, February 17, 1967 (Salt Lake City, Utah: Bureau of Mines, 1967).

[a] Copper as an integral part of the steel.

[b] Not determined.

TABLE 5-4, Part 1.   Amount of Dissolved Nonferrous Metal in Various Auto Parts

Parts	Weight (pounds)	Al Fraction	Al Pounds	Cu Fraction	Cu Pounds	Cr Fraction	Cr Pounds
Engine	454.5	0.000175	0.0796	0.0010	0.454	0.0038	1.73
Differential	153.5	0.00015	0.0030	0.0006	0.092	0.0016	0.245
Wheel covers and wheels	78.7	0.00005	0.0004	0.00015	0.0118	0.0003	0.0023(
Brake drums and cylinders	79.4	0.0002	0.0001	0.0012	0.0955	0.0032	0.254
Interior trim	21.1	0.0003	0.00633	0.0035	0.074	0.165	3.48
Mirrors, light covers	12.0	0.0003	0.0036	0.0035	0.042	0.165	1.98
Window frames	11.4	0.0003	0.00342	0.0035	0.040	0.165	1.89
Body trim and decoration	4.8	0.0003	0.00144	0.0035	0.018	0.165	0.792
Interior handles	3.6	0.0394	0.142	0.0045	0.0162	—	—
Exterior handles	4.2	0.0394	0.165	0.0045	0.0189	—	—
Transmission[a]	153.8	—	—	0.00015	0.00203	0.0003	0.0040(
Exterior trim and grill	15.5	—	—	0.002	0.035	0.002	0.031
Bumpers and trim	79.5	0.0002	0.0016	0.0011	0.0875	0.0022	0.175
Light iron	1136.8	0.0009	1.0241	0.0005	0.568	0.001	1.1368
Heavy iron	874.3			0.00015	0.131	0.0003	0.262
Total dissolved materials			1.45059		1.68593		11.98212

[a] Calculated on the assumption that a transmission contains 135 pounds heavy iron.

TABLE 5-4, Part 2.   Amount of Dissolved Nonferrous Metal in Various Auto Parts

Parts	Weight (pounds)	Pb Fraction	Pb Pounds	Mn Fraction	Mn Pounds	Mo Fraction	Mo Pounds
Engine	454.5	0.0037	1.68	0.0075	3.41	0.0003	0.136
Differential	153.5	0.0018	0.276	0.006	0.92	0.0003	0.0462
Wheel covers and wheels	78.7	0.00005	0.0004	0.004	0.32	0.0003	0.0236
Brake drums and cylinders	79.4	0.0037	0.294	0.008	0.64	0.0003	0.0238
Interior trim	21.1	—	—	0.003	0.0632	0.0003	0.00634
Mirrors, light covers	12.0	—	—	0.003	0.036	0.0003	0.00361
Window frames	11.4	—	—	0.003	0.034	0.0003	0.00342
Body trim and decoration	4.8	—	—	0.003	0.014	0.0003	0.00144
Interior handles	3.6	—	—	—	—	—	—
Exterior handles	4.2	—	—	—	—	—	—
Transmission[a]	153.8	—	—	0.004	0.54	0.0003	0.0462
Exterior trim and grill	15.5	0.0001	0.00155	0.006	0.093	—	—
Bumpers and trim	79.5	—	—	0.005	0.038	0.0003	0.0239
Light iron	1136.8	0.00002	0.00227	0.003	3.40	0.0003	0.342
Heavy iron	874.3	—	—	0.004	3.49	0.0003	0.272
Total dissolved materials			2.25422		12.9982		0.92851

[a] Calculated on the assumption that a transmission contains 135 pounds heavy iron.

TABLE 5-4, Part 3. Amount of Dissolved Nonferrous Metal in Various Auto Parts

Parts	Weight (pounds)	Ni Fraction	Ni Pounds	Sn Fraction	Sn Pounds	C Fraction	C Pounds
Engine	454.5	0.0010	0.4545	0.00016	0.0729	0.032	14.6
Differential	153.5	0.0008	0.123	0.0001	0.0154	0.018	2.76
Wheel covers and wheels	78.7	0.0004	0.0315	0.00007	0.00055	0.0031	0.244
Brake drums and cylinders	79.4	0.0012	0.0954	0.00018	0.00143	0.034	2.70
Interior trim	21.1	0.0029	0.0612	—	—	—	—
Mirrors, light covers	12.0	0.0029	0.0348	—	—	—	—
Window frames	11.4	0.0029	0.0331	—	—	—	—
Body trim and decoration	4.8	0.0029	0.0146	—	—	—	—
Interior handles	3.6	0.0085	0.0306	—	—	—	—
Exterior handles	4.2	0.0085	0.0357	—	—	—	—
Transmission[a]	153.8	0.00044	0.00595	0.00007	0.0009	0.0031	0.42
Exterior trim and grill	15.5	0.001	0.0155	—	—	—	—
Bumpers and trim	79.5	0.0227	2.	—	—	—	—
Light iron	1136.8	0.00063	0.717	0.00006	0.682	0.015	17.00
Heavy iron	874.3	0.00044	0.385	0.00007	0.613	0.0031	2.72
Total dissolved materials			4.8978		1.38618		40.444

[a] Calculated on the assumption that a transmission contains 135 pounds heavy iron.

TABLE 5-4, Part 4. Amount of Dissolved Nonferrous Metal in Various Auto Parts

Parts	Weight (pounds)	S Fraction	S Pounds	Si Fraction	Si Pounds
Engine	454.5	0.0009	0.409	0.02	9.1
Differential	153.5	0.00045	0.0691	0.019	2.92
Wheel covers and wheels	78.7	0.00005	0.0039	0.0006	0.00472
Brake drums and cylinders	79.4	0.0009	0.0715	0.0206	1.64
Interior trim	21.1	—	—	0.004	0.0843
Mirrors, light covers	12.0	—	—	0.004	0.048
Window frames	11.4	—	—	0.004	0.0457
Body trim and decoration	4.8	—	—	0.004	0.0192
Interior handles	3.6	—	—	0.0004	0.00144
Exterior handles	4.2	—	—	0.0004	0.00168
Transmission[a]	153.8	—	—	0.0006	0.081
Exterior trim and grill	15.5	—	—	—	—
Bumpers and trim	79.5	—	—	0.004	0.318
Light iron	1136.8	—	—	0.0005	0.568
Heavy iron	874.3	—	—	0.0006	0.525
Total dissolved materials			0.5535		15.357

[a] Calculated on the assumption that a transmission contains 135 pounds heavy iron.

Appendix B
Mathematical Structure of the Dismantling Model

The dismantling model was constructed as follows: Consider some specific part m, such as a generator. It contains materials (some of which are chemical elements) in two forms: first, as heterogeneous material (for example, a piece of copper wire, or a piece of brass) and second, as dissolved material (for example, copper dissolved in brass, or copper dissolved in steel). Let the superscript i denote a particular material (element or nonelement) and consider n of these materials as metals. Let c_m^i represent the material i in part m if i is a heterogeneous material only. If i is also a dissolved material, then part m will contain c_m^i plus g_m^i, that is, heterogeneous plus dissolved material. The units of c_m^i and g_m^i are pounds of material i in part m.

Let the superscript k denote the disposition of part m, where $k = 0$ signifies parts coming into the system, $k = 1$ signifies removal from the car body, $k = 2$ signifies disassembling for sale of the secondary materials, of which m is made, $k = 3$ signifies selling as is (that is, removing the part from the auto, but not disassembling the part), and $k = 4$ signifies disposing of the part as solid waste. Let x_m^k represent activities; that is x_m^k represents the total number of part m undergoing disposition k.[11]

Then,

$$(1) \quad x_m^k \geq 0 \qquad m = 1, 2, \ldots, 40$$
$$k = 0, 1, 2, 3, 4$$

Two particular parts, sets of light iron and sets of heavy iron ($m = 35$, 36), cannot be removed unless *all* other metallic parts are removed (because, by definition, they are the steel remaining in the car when all other parts have been removed). These so-called "parts" are in a sense

[11] The automobile is considered as having thirty-six basic parts as enumerated by Dean and Sterner. These parts and their compositions are listed in appendix A, table 5-2. In addition to the thirty-six basic components, the model also includes four "extras": sets of tires, sets of windows, sets of seats, and gasoline tanks, all of which must be removed prior to shredding. The extra parts are of course treated the same way as the basic thirty-six, except that they have no recovery value and are therefore disposed of as solid waste. Values of $m = 37, 38, 39, 40$ are used to denote these four extra parts.

artificial, in that they are left free after all the other parts have been removed. This is accounted for by a removal time of zero for the light iron and heavy iron sets.

(2) $x_{35}^1 \leq x_m^1$ $m = 1, 2, \ldots, 34$

(3) $x_{36}^1 \leq x_m^1$ $m = 1, 2, \ldots, 34$

Number balance considerations require that

(4) $x_m^1 = x_m^2 + x_m^3 + x_m^4$ $m = 1, 2, \ldots, 40$

Some parts always become solid waste.

(5) $x_m^0 = x_m^1 = x_m^4$ $m = 37, 38, 39, 40$

Let d represent the number of automobiles entering the system. Then

(6) $x_m^1 \leq x_m^0 = d$ $m = 1, 2, \ldots, 40$

Let y_i represent recovered (necessarily heterogeneous) metal in pounds of type i (considering n metals). Then

(7) $y_i = \sum\limits_{m=1}^{36} c_m^i x_m^2$ $i = 1, 2, \ldots, n$

The materials in the hulks leaving the system require another set of equations. These are material balance equations on the n metals plus a total of seven other materials of interest, including carbon, silicon, sulfur, rubber, glass, other combustibles, and other noncombustibles. If z^i represents the amount of material type i in one auto before dismantling, and v^i represents the amount of material of type i remaining in one auto after dismantling, then:

(8) $v^i = z^i - \sum\limits_{m=1}^{40} [c_m^i + g_m^i] x_m^3$

Therefore

(9) $v^i = z^i - \sum\limits_{m=1}^{36} [c_m^i + g_m^i] x_m^2 - \sum\limits_{m=1}^{36} [c_m^i + g_m^i] x_m^3 -$

$$\sum\limits_{m=1}^{40} [c_m^i + g_m^i] x_m^4$$

$$i = 1, 2, \ldots, n, n+1, \ldots, n+7$$

If u represents total tons solid waste produced per automobile, then

(10) $\sum\limits_{m=1}^{40} [c_m^i + g_m^i] x_m^4 = 2000\, u$

Let w represent total labor time in hours. Then if a_m represents the removal time for each part m and b_m represents the disassembling time for each part m then

(11) $\quad w = \sum\limits_{m=1}^{40} (a_m x_m^1 + b_m x_m^2)$

Further rows may be added to express whatever constraints the investigator is interested in studying. The objective is to maximize profit per automobile V, that is,

(12) $\quad \max V = -c_e w - c_{sw} u + \sum\limits_{m=1}^{36} p_m [c_m^i + g_m^i] x_m^3 +$

$$\sum\limits_{i=1}^{n} p_i y_i - c_a + c_b \sum\limits_{m=1}^{36} [c_m^i + g_m^i] x_m^0 / 2000$$

where c_{sw} represents cost of disposing of the solid waste in dollars per ton
$\quad c_e$ represents labor cost in dollars per hour
$\quad p_m$ represents the selling price of unassembled part m
$\quad p_i$ represents the selling price of metal i
$\quad c_a$ represents the cost of obtaining a deregistered automobile
$\quad c_b$ represents the price obtained for a hulk in units of $/ton

The equations above formally describe a mathematical model of automobile dismantling as conventionally practiced.

The difficulties of using a standard linear programming solution algorithm for a problem that has some variables restricted to integer values are well known. While they cannot be simply dismissed, the extent of the problem created by this approximation method is related to the particular mixed integer programming problem being solved. For example, if the integer values being found are very large, the errors become very small.

In the case of the automobile dismantling model, the complications created are considerably reduced by a special set of circumstances. The major constraint is that the sum of five nonferrous impurities be less than or equal to some particular weight percent of the dismantled hulk. The metals are copper, chrome, nickel, molybdenum, and tin. Four of the five metals occur mostly in solid solution in the steel body of the car. Copper is present, however, in heterogeneous form; it is also a valuable metal. Thus as the constraint is parametrically varied to lower and lower tolerable levels of the sum of the five contaminants, it is the copper-bearing parts that are removed, rather than parts which contain some mixture of all the metals. The parts are removed in order of decreasing marginal profit (which, of course, actually goes negative). Because of this unusual circumstance, the continuous solution to the mixed-integer problem is a reasonable approximation to the correct integer-valued solution. This situation seems to prevail except for the very lowest levels of contamination which in fact are not economically practical to achieve.

This conclusion is demonstrated by computer runs in which the contraint is parametrically varied. An examination of the activity levels at each contamination constraint level reveals a series of zero and one activity levels for the removal of various parts (for one car entering the system) and only one activity level which is fractional. At the next lower (more severe) constraint level, the previous noninteger activity moves either to a large fractional number or else to one. In the latter case, an activity removal step which had previously been zero valued starts being performed at a fractional level. This pattern prevails down to very low constraint levels, at which point the solution pattern changes, and becomes a series of zeroes, ones, and a number of fractional removal levels. It is at this point that the noninteger solution starts becoming a poor approximation to the true optimum. However, the experiments run clearly indicate that this is at a constraint level that would not occur in practice because of the loss of profits to the dismantler.

Thus for the feasible space of the greatest interest, while the solution may indicate that a fraction of a part should be removed, if a true integer solution were obtained, it would apparently be the next larger integer above the fractional value indicated by the linear programming solution.

6

Hulk Transportation and Processing

HULK TRANSPORT

After dismantling, automobile hulks are shipped to a central processor on large trucks that carry from six to forty hulks at a time. A device called a flattener flattens a hulk 5 feet high down to 1 foot. With flattening, as many as forty hulks can be loaded on one tractor trailer; without it, the truck can hold only six hulks. In contrast, deregistered automobiles are shipped to the dismantler one at a time via tow truck or other small truck.

Our observations in the field indicate that the average number of flattened hulks being carried was about fifteen to twenty-five, despite the potential for larger shipments. The reason for this is not clear; there may not be a large number of hulks available at a single location, or highway load limits may keep the number down.

Since there is an appreciable cost in flattening (about $4 per hulk), a dismantler has to make an economic decision as to whether or not he will flatten his hulks before shipping. If he does not choose to flatten, shipping costs go up. If, on the other hand, he flattens the hulks, the shipping cost per hulk will be lower, but the cost of flattening will have to be added to it.

In studying transportation costs for auto hulks this work utilized the results of Adams[1] which are based on data gathered from an August 1970 Bureau of Mines survey and from the U.S. Department of Commerce (1968). Since practically all hulks are transported by truck, the transportation cost per hulk is a function of the number of hulks carried

---

[1] See R. L. Adams, "An Economic Analysis of the Junk Automobile Problem," unpublished Ph.D. dissertation, Department of Economics, University of Illinois, 1972, chapter IV.

per truckload and the distance the hulks are shipped. Adams found that the number of hulks per truckload can range from one unflattened hulk on a small dump truck to as many as forty flattened hulks on a large flatbed truck. To develop a relation between cost and miles shipped, the Commerce cost data were inflated (by means of the wholesale price index) to make the 1968 data comparable with the August 1970, Bureau of Mines data. Adams found that for truckloads of flattened hulks, the cost can be approximated by the following regression equation:

(1) $\ln y = 2.05 + 0.59 \ln x$

where y represents cost in dollars per truckload and x represents miles shipped. The variance removed by the log-log regression was 0.927 and the standard deviation for the 0.59 was about 0.04. Adams also discovered that:

1. The costs per truckload of unflattened hulks as a function of miles shipped also agreed quite closely with equation (1);
2. While the truckloads of flattened hulks varied from twenty to forty hulks per load, the cost per truckload versus miles hauled all fell around the estimated equation values.

The August 1970 survey of shredded scrap producers indicated that in 1969, 60 percent of the hulks arrived in an unflattened condition in trucks carrying from five to eight hulks per load.[2] A basic assumption is that six unflattened cars will be shipped per truckload. Thus, it can be shown that equation (1) implies[3]

(2)   cost per car $= (1/6) \, (7.78 \, x^{0.59})$

If cars are flattened, this cost must be added to the shipping cost if a comparison is to be made between shipping unflattened versus flattened hulks. Adams calculated that the cost of flattening a hulk is $4.15 per

---

[2] *Ibid.*, p. 199.
[3] It should be noted that equation (1) implies that the "power method" is being used in the calculation of transportation costs. This can be demonstrated as follows: first, exponentiate both sides of equation (1) and use the value of e to obtain:

$$Y = 7.78 \, x^{0.59}$$

Next, let (x_1, y_1) and (x_2, y_2) be two pairs of points satisfying equation (1). Then dividing one expression by the other, obtain:

$$\frac{Y_2}{Y_1} = \frac{7.78 \, x_2^{0.59}}{7.78 \, x_1^{0.59}} = \left(\frac{x_2}{x_1} \right)^{0.59}$$

This demonstrates that the power method is implicitly being used in the calculation of transportation costs.

car. Adams' cost calculations for flattening made a number of assumptions.[4] The cost of shipment per flattened hulk is

$$\text{cost per car} = 4.15 + (1/N) \ (7.78 \ x^{0.59})$$

where N represents the number of hulks shipped per truckload.

The shipping method used will be the one that minimizes cost, that is:

(3) $\text{cost per car} = \min \ \{(1/6) \ 7.78 \ x^{0.59}, 4.15 + (1/N) \ 7.78 \ x^{0.59}\}$

Equation (3) is used in the model. The value of x for which the optimal mode of transportation shifts from no flattening to flattening is about 10 miles, assuming $N = 40$. In the operation of the total hulk processing model, care was taken to parametrically vary N to determine its effect on the model's predictions.

To reiterate the purpose of developing equation (3), the hulk transport section of the model assumes that hulks are produced by dismantlers located in the same place as the population, and that all hulks are being sent to one central processing location. Thus the cost of a hulk to the central processor varies with the distance from the dismantler to the central processor. Equation (3) calculates this shipment cost.

COSTS OF PROCESSING HULKS INTO STEEL SCRAP

This section discusses the development of hulk processing equipment cost estimates. The principal virtue of the costing procedure developed is that it provides for easily varying prices and other parameters as the data base improves. Yet, the formulation of the model is explicit, and the methodology can therefore be effectively criticized and improved by knowledgeable representatives of the steel scrap industry. It is for this reason that the costing procedure itself is discussed in detail.

There are currently four major types of equipment used to process steel scrap: the incinerator, the baler, the shear, and the shredder. A literature search and numerous discussions with dealers revealed that published cost data are scarce.[5] Therefore the required data on investment costs and labor requirements were obtained from manufacturers

---

[4] Adams' assumptions were:
   a. The flattener is portable and can operate at a rate of 20 hulks per hour.
   b. A flattener will flatten hulks for half of the standard 2080-hour year. The remaining time will be spent in moving from place to place.
   c. All labor will be paid on the basis of a full standard year.
   d. The project is expected to have a 10-year life.
   e. A federal income tax of 48 percent and a state income tax of 5 percent are assumed.

[5] For example, John G. Clement, Resource Planning Institute, Cambridge, Mass., telephone communications, March 1972 and October 1972.

and scrap processors. A limited sampling of baler and shear manufacturers was performed, since for both of these items investment costs are relatively small, and the production of these machines is a mature enterprise. That is, competitive market forces assure a fair measure of cost agreement among different manufacturers. See tables 6-1 and 6-2, and figures 6-1 to 6-6.

TABLE 6-1. Capital Costs for Baling Presses[a]

del	Manufacturer	Estimated input (and output) capacity in gross tons/hr.	No. of men required for operation	Estimated purchase price in thousands of dollars	Estimated installation cost in thousands of dollars	Total investment in thousands of dollars	Investment as thousands of dollars per gross ton per hour output	Total horsepower installed
A	1	1.5	1	22	24	46	30.6	—
B	11	1.5–3	—	25	25	50	22.2	30
C	11	3.5–5	—	50	29	79	16.6	75
D	11	10–15	—	100	38	138	11.0	155
E	1	7–9	3	166	50	217	27.2	128
F	1	14.5	3	176	51	224	15.4	228
G	1	16.3	3	200	55	225	13.8	228
H	1	20.5	3	210	57	267	13.0	328
	1	22.8	3	297	73	371	16.3	428
	1	27.1	4	439	98	537	19.8	528
	1	37.3	4	530	114	644	17.3	628

[a] Data as of June 1972 from interviews with scrap processors and equipment manufacturers.

TABLE 6-2. Capital Costs for Baler-Shear (Guillotine Shear)[a]

aler-ear del	Estimated input (and output) capacity in gross tons/hr.	No. of men required for operation	Estimated purchase price in thousands of dollars	Estimated installation cost in thousands of dollars	Total investment in thousands of dollars	Investment as thousands of dollars per gross ton per hour output	Total horsepower installed
A	6–8	3	140	45	185	26.4	108
B	6–8	3	150	46	196	28.0	208
C	7–9	4	174	51	225	28.1	208
D	7–9	4	184	53	237	29.6	308
E	7–9	3	160	48	208	26.0	108
F	7–9	3	170	50	220	27.5	208
G	7–9	4	181	52	233	29.1	208
H	7–9	4	191	54	245	30.6	308
I	8–10	4	173	51	224	24.9	208
J	8–10	4	183	53	236	26.2	308
K	10–12	4	191	54	245	22.2	308
L	11–13	4	230	61	291	24.2	308
M	12–15	4	283	71	354	26.2	308
N	14–17	5	322	77	399	25.8	408
O	20–22	5	446	117	563	26.8	608
P	20–22	5	420	95	515	24.6	608
Q	25–30	6	650	136	786	28.6	1030

[a] Data as of June 1972 from interviews with scrap processors and equipment manufacturers.

However, neither of these assumptions appears valid for shredders. Figure 6-1 reveals significant variations in the estimated costs of buying and installing a shredder. As this problem became apparent during the

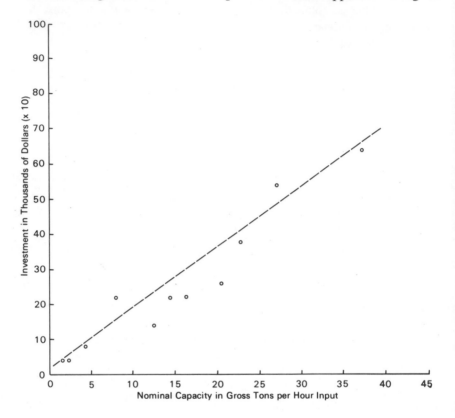

FIGURE 6-1.   Baler investment data. Investment costs in thousands of dollars, including installation expenses as a function of nominal capacity in gross tons per hour. Equation is $Y = 17500.00\ (X) + 20000.00$ where Y represents investment in dollars and X represents nominal capacity in gross tons per hour.

study, special attention was focused on obtaining as much shredder data as possible.[6] As a result, six shredder operators and eight shredder manufacturers were contacted. Most provided some data, usually with

---

[6] Two important sources of published shredder data costs are Adams, "An Economic Analysis" and C. Wilkinson, Newell Manufacturing Co., San Antonio, Texas, letter to J. W. Sawyer, June 7, 1972. Adams developed four hypothetical shredders and presented estimated cost data for them. His data sources are personal contacts and manufacturers' reports. Newell is a large shredder manufacturer who has written an article and several brochures on shredder costs.

the proviso that the source not be revealed. All these data are displayed in table 6-3 and figures 6-1 to 6-6.[7]

Cost and manpower data for incinerators and cyclone separators (cyclone separators are used to reduce particulate emissions from shredders) were more difficult to obtain. The most well-known estimates of auto hulk incinerator costs are those of Chindgren, Dean, and Sterner[8]

[7] Shredder cost data were developed on the basis that a car prepared for a shredder weighs about 1 gross ton. If 75 percent of input is recovered, a 100 gross ton input shredder would have a capacity of 75 gross ton output, or about 84 net tons. This situation is confused by the fact that both scrap operations and shredder companies are quite ambiguous about capacities. Question: "What is the capacity of this unit?" Answer: "53 tons per hour." When neither net tons nor gross tons are specified, and neither is a statement as to whether it is input or output tonnage, the answer leaves room for more questions, most of which the dealer is not really eager to answer. The situation is further complicated by the fact that shredder manufacturers want to give selling costs, not installed cost. In cases where both selling cost and installed cost were available, the factor seemed to be about 2.0, and this factor was used when complete data were not available. Manpower requirements were obtained by interviewing shredder operators only.

[8] U.S. Department of the Interior, Bureau of Mines, *Construction and Testing of a Junk Auto Incinerator*, by C. J. Chindgren, K. C. Dean, and J. W. Sterner, Bureau of Mines Solid Waste Research Program, Technical Progress Report 21, 1970.

TABLE 6-3.   Capital Costs for Shredders[a]

Shredder	Total manpower	Number of men to run	Number of men to maintain	Input in gross tons/hr.	Estimated output in gross tons/hr.	Estimated installed cost in million dollars	Investment as thousands of dollars per gross ton/hr. output
1	31	—	—	110	84.3	3.5	41.5
2	28	22	6	94	72.0	3.0	41.7
3	—	—	—	12–15	10.7	0.35	34.0
4	—	—	—	20–25	17.2	0.75	43.5
5	—	—	—	20–25	17.2	0.825	46.9
6	—	—	—	28	21.4	0.65	30.4
7	—	—	—	112	85.8	2.0	23.3
8	—	—	—	17	13.0	0.5	38.4
9	—	—	—	34	26.6	1.25	48.2
10	—	—	—	56	42.9	1.8	42.0
11	8	—	—	30	23.0	0.8	34.8
12	—	—	—	22	16.8	0.6	35.7
13	—	—	—	17	13.0	0.2	15.4
14	—	—	—	48	36.8	0.54	14.7
15	—	—	—	84	64.3	1.0	15.5
16	10	8	2	29	22.2	1.0	45.2
17	35	—	—	100	76.6	—	—
18	12	—	—	20	15.3	—	—
19	10	8	2	18	13.8	—	—
20	12	9	3	55	42.1	—	—

[a] Data as of 1972 from interviews with shredder operators and manufacturers.

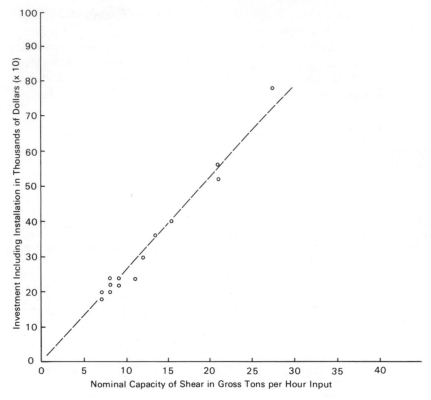

Investment Including Installation in Thousands of Dollars (x 10)

FIGURE 6-2.   Data for baler-shears. Investment costs in thousands of dollars,
including installation expenses, as a function of nominal capacity in gross tons
per hour.

of the U.S. Bureau of Mines. Their study indicated an investment cost
of $22,000 for a 50 car-per-day incinerator. However, a scrap proc-
essor[9] was interviewed who recently (1972) built a 100 car-per-day
incinerator, and the cost of that incinerator far exceeded the cost which
would have been suggested by the above-mentioned Bureau of Mines
study, performed in 1968. This single 1972 data point appeared to be
the best estimate of actual costs that would be incurred.[10]

The calculation of investment cost for incinerators of differing capaci-

[9] Personal interview at company offices with J. Zuckerman, Zuckerman Co., Inc.,
Winchester, Va., June 2, 1972.

[10] Late in the course of the study, yet another scrap processor was found who
had built a "pollution-free" incinerator. His reported costs were in line with those
calculated herein, rather than the Bureau of Mines data.

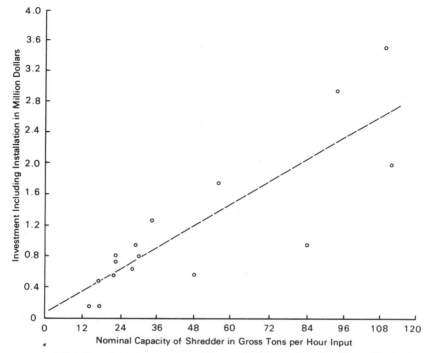

FIGURE 6-3. Investment costs in millions of dollars for shredders. Data obtained from both shredder operators and shredder sellers. Equation is $Y = 73300.00 + 23600.00 \ (X)$ where Y represents investment in dollars and X represents input capacity in gross tons per hour.

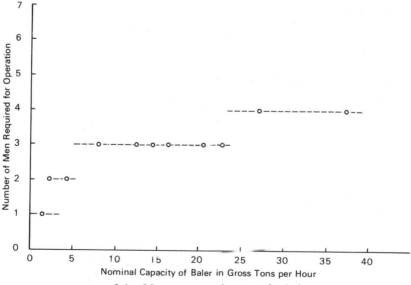

FIGURE 6-4. Manpower requirements for balers.

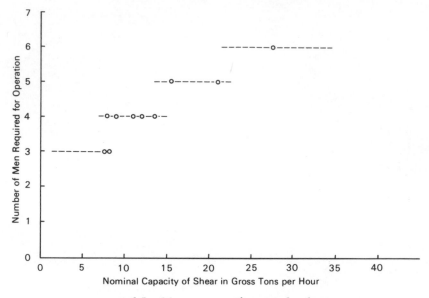

FIGURE 6-5.   Manpower requirements for shears.

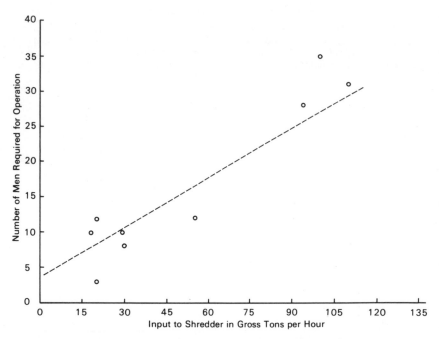

FIGURE 6-6.   Manpower requirements for shredders. Data obtained by plant trip interviews and by some telephone interviews. Equation for line is, $Y = 3 + 0.26 (X)$ where Y is manpower requirement and X is gross tons input to shredder.

ties was accomplished by using the well-known power method.[11] Briefly, the power method asserts that

$$(4) \quad \frac{C_i}{C_j} = \left[\frac{q_i}{q_j} \right]^k$$

where C_i, C_j represent the investment costs of the ith and j^{th} plants, respectively; q_i and q_j are the corresponding capacities; and k is a constant between 0 and 1 for the particular type of equipment under consideration. If k is not known,[12] a value of 0.7 is assumed, since it has been found to be a good approximation for widely varying types of equipment. The reported cost of the 50 car-per-day Bureau of Mines unit was $22,000. Using the power method, the calculated cost is $140,000. At least some of this disparity is caused by the inflation of the past 4 years.[13] The remainder of the disparity must await further research for resolution.

It was assumed that labor requirements for incinerators are directly proportional to capacity. Knowledge of the manpower requirements for the particular incinerator visited allowed an approximate estimate of labor requirements for incinerators of varying capacities.

Interviews with several shredder operators indicated that cyclone separator costs were in the $50,000–100,000 range, with no exact figures forthcoming. To clarify this situation, A. H. Nickolaus,[14] calculated typical cyclone separator costs. The design basis was 7.5 tons per hour of dust entering the unit and 95 percent collection efficiency.[15] A 100 hulk-per-hour shredder is estimated to produce about 1 ton of dust per hour or about 20 pounds per car. Unfortunately, there is no way of being certain of the 20-pound per car factor.[16] Even a large discrepancy

---

[11] See M. S. Peters and K. D. Timmerhaus, *Plant Design and Economics for Chemical Engineers* (McGraw-Hill, 1971), p. 122.

[12] The value of k can be found only by detailed cost calculations for the type of plant involved over a range of sizes.

[13] In 1968 the Department of Commerce Composite Construction Cost Index was about 103 (see *Statistical Abstract of the United States: 1972*, 93rd ed., 1972, p. 677), while the same index for 1972 can be estimated from the data given as about 142 for 1972. Thus, the expected cost of the U.S. Bureau of Mines unit would be at least (142/102) (22,000), or about $30,000. The discrepancy between this and the cost of the unit actually built using the Bureau of Mines basic design seems very large.

[14] Telephone communication with Andrew H. Nickolaus, E.I. du Pont de Nemours & Co., Inc., Victoria, Texas, July 1972.

[15] The design basis was 7.5 tons/hour since the cost estimate was made well before data were obtained which suggested that 1 top/hour would be a better basis for the required calculations.

[16] This is a consensus figure derived from interviews with shredder operators during the study. It is an average figure for the mix of hulks currently (1972) being fed to shredders.

in the assumed level of dust generation has little effect on the model, since the sensitivity of total processing costs to cyclone separator costs is nil.[17] The estimated cost was \$47,500 (1972 prices). Installation costs would probably double this, for a total cost of \$95,000. Nickolaus reported that a good scale-up factor to use would be 0.7. That is,

$$(5) \quad \frac{C_i}{\$95,000} = \left[\frac{q_i}{15,000 \text{ lbs./hr.}} \right]^{0.7}$$

where C_i represents the cost of ith unit and q_i is the corresponding capacity. This equation was approximated by a straight line over the range of interest. The equation for the line is

$$(6) \quad C = 37,000 + 4.29 \, q$$

where C represents investment cost in dollars and q represents the input capacity of the cyclone separator in gross tons of dust per year (2080-hour year). In accordance with observed practice, manpower requirements were assumed to be constant and small and were estimated to be 0.05 man hour per operating hour. The capacity utilization factor was assumed to be 100 percent, since this type of equipment is very reliable. However, costs were calculated as a function of the capacity utilization factor of the shredder because when the shredder is incapacitated, the cyclone separator is also.

A unit such as this should last 15–20 years and require only a small amount of maintenance (about 2 percent). It should effectively remove all particles larger than 10–20 microns.[18] Obviously, its collection efficiency varies with particle density as well as other variables; however, an assumption of 95 percent removal seems very conservative for particles over 1/100 of an inch.[19]

These assumptions are consistent with observations at the six shredding plants visited and with the comments of the owners and operators. The dust particles are, to the eye, relatively large, and a well-designed

---

[17] Suppose (a highly radical supposition) that the operating cost of a cyclone separator is \$5 per gross ton of dust rather than \$1.97. Assuming 20 pounds of dust per car, \$5 per gross ton implies a cost of about 12.5 cents per car. This is about 1.5 percent of the cost of operating a shredder. Of course it would be a far higher percentage of the profits from running a shredder.

The required cyclone separator would be about 6 feet in diameter and would handle 17,000 cubic feet/minute of incoming air. It was assumed that the air would enter through a pipe which would be 1½ feet in diameter and 100 feet in length. These requirements, which corresponded well with what was observed on visits to shredder installations, implied a 40 horsepower motor and a \$47,500 cost (1972 prices).

[18] A micron is a millionth of a meter; thus 10 microns is about 0.0004 inch.

[19] See John H. Perry (ed.), *Chemical Engineers' Handbook*, 3rd ed. (McGraw-Hill, 1950), pp. 1026–1027.

cyclone separator has an exit air stream which appears to be free of dust. This illusion would, of course, be eliminated by a careful investigation with modern equipment.[20]

COSTING PROCEDURE

The costing procedure that was adopted is thoroughly discussed in such texts as Peters and Timmerhaus[21] and is often used in the chemical industry. Three types of costs are considered: fixed, semivariable, and variable. Fixed costs are independent of the production rate for a process of a given size; amortization is a fixed cost, since it must be paid regardless of output. Variable costs are related only to production rate; raw materials costs are variable costs since in most cases a doubling of plant output will result in a doubling of the consumption of the required raw materials. Labor, on the other hand, is a good example of a semivariable cost—a cost that is partially fixed and partially related to plant output. This is the case since even at very low levels of output some labor is required.

Variable costs for the five types of scrap processing units and for open burning are listed in table 6-4. These data were obtained as follows:

[20] A side remark: asbestos particles from automobile brake linings flake off during usage and are thus present in city air. Are they coarse, thus allowing their collection as solid waste in the cyclone separator, or do they escape into the air via the separator? If the latter is true, this process could be a large source of asbestos particles in city air. This should be checked by the Environmental Protection Agency.

[21] Peters and Timmerhaus, *Plant Design*.

TABLE 6-4. Variable Inputs and Nonproduct Outputs (Residuals) Associated with Steel Scrap Processing Equipment

Factor	Type of process				
	Incineration	Baler	Shear	Shredder	Cyc. Sep.
electricity (kWh gr. ton input)	3.00	10.20	6.40	42.5	5.97
water (gal./gr. ton proc.)	10.00	700.00	400.00	240.00	0.00
gas (1000 cu. ft./car proc.)	0.08	0.00	0.00	0.00	0.00
kerosene (gal./car proc.)	7.00	0.00	0.00	0.00	0.00
diesel fuel (gal./car proc.)	0.00	0.00	0.00	1.75	0.00
carb. monoxide (lbs./gr. ton proc.)	3.61	0.00	0.00	0.00	0.00
carb. dioxide (lbs./gr. ton proc.)	3.61	0.00	0.00	0.00	0.00
nitrogen oxides (lbs./gr. ton proc.)	0.36	0.00	0.00	0.00	0.00
particulates (lbs./gr. ton proc.)	0.21	0.00	0.00	20.00	0.00
capacity utilization as a fraction of capacity	0.90	0.90	0.90	0.90	0.90
O_2 per car burned (lbs.)	0.90	0.00	0.00	0.00	0.00

1. Kerosene requirements for open burning are from interviews with dealers
2. Water requirements for shears and shredders are from Adams[22]
3. Water requirements for balers were scaled up from water requirements for shears, assuming that a constant amount of water per horsepower/ton is required
4. Electricity requirements for shredders as reported by a number of scrap processors are 28.0–33.0 kilowatt hours/net ton product; Adams[23] states shredder electricity requirements as 44.0 kilowatt hours/net ton[24] (a value of 29.0 was used in the model); calculated supply and elasticity of supply are quite insensitive to the value chosen.
5. Electricity requirements for cyclone separations are from Nicholaus[25]
6. The required water cost data for industrial users of this size class (which includes sewage costs) were obtained from the Philadelphia Water Department
7. The information utilized was obtained from interviews with scrap processors

The costing procedure employed is now described. Investment costs were assumed to be linearly related to capacity; that is:

$$(7) \quad C_k = a_k + b_k Q_k$$

where k represents the unit under consideration, C^k its investment cost in 1972 dollars, a_k and b_k are constants (in all cases a_k was effectively zero), and Q_k its nominal capacity in gross tons per hour. In the case of the baler and the baler-shear, the output capacity equals the input capacity almost exactly, whereas in the case of the shredder only about 70–80 percent of the feed is actually converted to useful ferrous scrap. Therefore cost equations for the shredder are given in terms of both Q_3^{input} and Q_3^{output}. The factor used was 1 ton input equals 0.766 tons output, this being the average factor found from the shredder operators reporting information on conversion factors for the shredding operation. Using an assumed relationship of the form of (7) above, regression analyses indicated:

---

[22] R. L. Adams, "An Economic Analysis of the Junk Automobile Problem," unpublished Ph.D. dissertation, Department of Economics, University of Illinois, 1972.

[23] *Ibid.*

[24] Adams does not indicate whether input or output. However, 29.0 kilowatt hours per net ton output is equivalent to about 39 kilowatt hours per net ton input.

[25] Telephone communication with Andrew H. Nickolaus, E.I. du Pont de Nemours & Co., Inc., July 1972.

(8) $C_1 - 16,710\,Q_1$ (baler); r-squared 0.925, t-statistic 10.5

(9) $C_2 = 26,670\,Q_2$ (baler-shear); r-squared 0.975, t-statistic 24.1

(10) $C_3 = 23,309\,Q_3$ input (shredder); r-squared 0.918, t-statistic 6.0

(11) $C_3 = 30,430\,Q_3$ output (shredder); statistics same as above

In all cases, equipment resale values were assumed to be zero, since no data were available. The model is general, however, and allows for their incorporation.

A linear relationship was also assumed to hold between manpower requirements and nominal capacity for the shredder. Two equations were derived, one for the case where the capacity of the shredder was rated in terms of gross tons per hour input, one for the case where the capacity of the shredder was rated in terms of gross tons per hour output capacity (the latter of course is the more usual assessment of capacity).[26]

(12) $M_3 = 0.27\,Q_3^{\text{input}} + 3$; r-squared 0.967, t-statistic 3.4 for
constant, 20.3 for capacity

(13) $M_3 = 0.33\,Q_3^{\text{output}} + 4$; r-squared 0.962, t-statistic 4.4 for
constant, 18.9 for capacity

However, in the case of the baler and shear, figure 6-2 demonstrates that a linear relationship does not hold between manpower requirements and nominal capacity. The data indicate that manpower requirements for balers and shears are constant over different ranges of capacity. Thus, these integer step relationships were used for the determination of manpower requirements.

Three typically sized units for each of the six types of scrap processing equipment were selected. These choices were based on the general sense of the industry gained from numerous visits to scrap processors. The chosen capacities and their corresponding manpower requirements are listed in table 6-5. In the case of the shredder, manpower requirements are those given by equation (9) minus an estimate of maintenance labor, since maintenance is costed separately. For the baler and shear, manpower requirements are based on visual inspection of figures 6-4 to 6-6. Manpower requirements for incinerators and cyclone separators were previously discussed. The routine aspects of the cost calculations are included as a footnote.[27]

---

[26] When these regressions were run, a constraint was included that ensured that the constants in the equations would be integer values.

[27] Let INT represent the interest rate, C_k the cost of the kth unit of specified capacity, S_k the resale value of the kth unit of specified capacity, R_k the amortiza-

An examination of the calculated data demonstrated that, if other variables operate within their normal ranges, the most important determinant of costs is the capacity utilization factor. Even in those cases in which idle labor is assumed to cost nothing, the variation in cost with capacity utilization is quite large. For a shredder operation, idle labor

---

tion per year required to pay for the equipment, and LT the lifetime of the machine in years. Fixed costs—maintenance cost (MC), operating supplies (OSC), and taxes and insurance (TI)—are now calculated. Let

$MFACT$ represent a maintenance factor

$OSFACT$ represent an operating supplies factor

$TAXINS$ represent a taxes and insurance factor

Then:

$$MC = (MFACT) \, (C_k - S_k)$$
$$OSC = (OSFACT) \, (MC)$$
$$TI = (TAXINS) \, (C_k - S_k)$$

where $MFACT$, $OSFACT$, $TAXINS$ are fractions between 0 and 1. Based on the discussion in Peters and Timmerhaus (footnote 11), the following values were used: $MFACT$ = .10 for shredder; .06 for other units; $OSFACT$ = .20; $TAXINS$ = .02. (All shredder operators visited agreed that maintenance costs are high compared with other scrap equipment.)

The calculation of labor costs (LC) is complicated by the problem of estimating labor costs when the machine is idle. Three cases were considered:

1. When the machine is idle, labor costs are 0:

$$LC = (LABORR) \, (MPW) \, (HRSPYR) \, (UTI)$$

where $LABORR$ is the labor rate ($/hour), MPW is the number of men per year required for operation, $HRSPYR$ is hours per year (assumed to be 2080), and UTI is the capacity utilization of the unit in question. An equivalent assumption is that labor can be employed at the same profit level elsewhere in the plant when the machine is down.

2. When the machine is idle, labor costs drop to half their normal rate:

$$LC = (LABORR) \, (MPW) \, (HYSPYR) \, [(1 + UTI)/2]$$

Equivalently, half the labor can be employed elsewhere at the same profit level.

3. When the machine is idle, labor costs must be fully charged to operating expenses for the machines:

$$LC = (LABORR) \, (MPW) \, (HRSPYR)$$

Supervision Costs (SC) and labor benefits (LB) are assumed to be fixed percentages of labor costs:

$$SC = (SUPVIS) \, (LC)$$

$$LB = (LABBEN) \, (LC)$$

where $SUPVIS$, $LABBEN$ are fractions between 0 and 1. Again, based on the discussion in Peters and Timmerhaus, we have assumed that $SUPVIS$ = .17, $LABBEN$ = .33. Plant overhead and administration costs (OAC) are computed as follows:

$$OAC = OVADM \, (LC + LB + SC + MC)$$

where $OVADM$ is a fraction between 0 and 1 and is assumed equal to .75 in this study. It should be noted that all of these parameters (e.g., $OVADM$, $SUPVIS$)

seems just that—idle labor. If idle labor is totally nonproductive, a decrease in capacity utilization factor from 90 to 60 percent indicates an increase in cost from $6.85 to $11.40, or an increase of $4.55 per gross ton output.

These changes in cost as a function of capacity utilization factor and cost of idle labor are important because, while balers and baler-shears are highly reliable and operate 90–95 percent of the time, the shredder is a temperamental and unreliable device. These facts are known by

---

can be varied at will by the programmer as the data base improves. Thus, average fixed and semivariable costs (APQ) are calculated using the following formula:

$$APQ = \frac{(LC + LB + SC + OAC + MC + OSC + TI)}{(HRSPYR)\,(CAP)\,[UTI\,(k)]}$$

where CAP is nominal capacity in gross tons per hour input of auto hulks.

Labor rate and utility were varied to determine the sensitivity of average costs to the various parameters.

Open burning was not considered in detail since it is outlawed in most areas and its fixed and semivariable costs, which essentially consist of labor and land rental costs, are small. In the case of the cyclone separator, labor costs are so low that they are insensitive to the assumption made.

The costs used in the model do not include amortization, since short-term elasticities of supply were being sought. That is, the capacities were constrained to those of the existing equipment in Philadelphia. If new plant construction were to be considered, then amortization should be included. Using the capital recovery factor,

$$R_k = (C_k - S_k)\,\frac{INT\,(1.0 + INT)^{LT}}{(1.0 + INT)^{LT} - 1.0}$$

costs appropriate for making decisions about installing new equipment in the region can be obtained.

$$APQ_{\text{long run}} = APQ + \frac{R_k}{(HRSPYR)\,(CAP)\,[UTI(k)]}$$

Using a 12 percent interest rate and a lifetime of 10 years for all equipment, the following costs result:

Incineration:	$5.01 per gross ton
Baling:	$4.39 per gross ton input or output
Shearing:	$5.27 per gross ton input or output
Shredding:	$7.43 per gross ton input
	$9.70 per gross ton output
Dust collection:	$4.12 per gross ton of dust input

The model was not run with these costs. However, it is clear from the mathematics of the model and the sense of how the model responds to changes in scrap prices that, given a difference between the price of No. 1 Heavy Melting and No. 2 Bundles of greater than $10 per gross ton, and given a price of No. 1 Heavy Melting of about $35 per gross ton (or more), there will be an economic motivation for increasing shredding capacity up to the level at which no more automobiles are available. This scenario is now being realized in the Philadelphia region.

TABLE 6-5. Fixed and Semivariable Cost Data and Other Data Necessary for Making Scrap Processing Cost Estimates

Factor considered	Process				
	Incinerator	Baler	Shear	Shredder	Cycl separ
Fixed component of investment in thousands of dollars (from equations 8, 9, 11)	80.00	00.00	00.00	00.00	37.
Incremental investment in dollars per gross ton output per year additional capacity (from equations 8, 9, 11)	4.81	8.04	12.8	14.60	4.
Relative nominal input capacity of unit in gross tons per hour (see figure 6-7)					
Low	6.00	10.00	10.00	30.00	2.
Medium	12.00	20.00	20.00	70.00	5.
High	24.00	30.00	30.00	120.00	9.
Normal manpower requirements for different nominal input capacities					
Low	1.00	3.00	4.00	8.00	0.
Medium	2.00	3.00	5.00	16.00	0.
High	4.00	4.00	6.00	27.00	0.

dealers and equipment manufacturers alike. Stone found the average capacity utilization factor to be 65 percent in a 1968 study.[28] In the same study Stone reported that the capacity utilization factor of balers and shears was 89 percent and 93 percent respectively. However, a 1971 study performed for the Bureau of Mines and reported by Battelle[29] indicated a capacity utilization factor of about 90 percent for shredders. Observations made in the course of this study suggest that the utility of a shredder varies with time—and the particular shredder being used. For some shredders that were observed, the capacity utilization was estimated to be well over 90 percent; that is, almost 10 operating days every 2 weeks. In other cases, downtime appeared to account for 2 days per week, or a capacity utilization factor of 60 percent.[30]

[28] See Ralph J. Stone, *Resource Reclamation: Yard Efficiency, A Preliminary Study of Scrapping Processes and Site Planning*, Report to the U.S. Department of the Interior, Bureau of Mines, Grant No. GO 180529 (SWD-20) (Ralph J. Stone and Co., Engineers, 1969).

[29] See W. J. Regan, R. W. James, and T. J. McLeer, *Final Report on Identification of Opportunities for Increased Recycling of Ferrous Solid Waste*, Report by the Battelle Memorial Institute to the Scrap Metal Research and Education Foundation of the Institute of Scrap Iron and Steel, Inc., 1971.

[30] One shredder dealer visited claimed that he had knowledge that nearly every major shredder installation in the United States had experienced at least one motor burn-out caused by the repeated shock impulses from the impact of the hammers

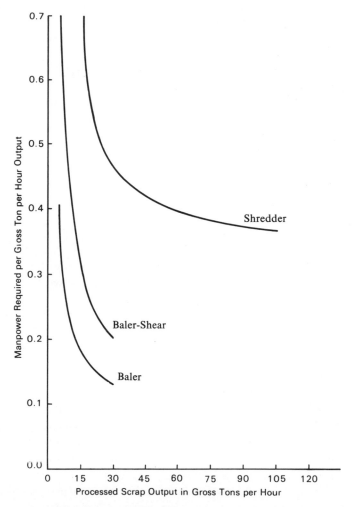

FIGURE 6-7. Manpower requirements for scrap processing equipment expressed as manpower per gross ton/hour output capacity which is equivalent to man hours per gross ton scrap produced. (Curves for baler and shear are idealized. Actual functions contain discontinuities.)

on the auto bodies. Assume, for the moment, that he is partially correct. The replacement of a 2000–3000 horsepower motor is not a minor repair for a company with a few employees and a small capital base. Moreover, one places more credence in the story when he has seen the specially designed magnetic clutches as well as the diesel engine—V-belt drive systems which are often used to attenuate shock impulses.

Based on the methodology and data presented above, processing costs were estimated using the following assumptions:
1.   Ninety percent capacity utilization factor for all equipment
2.   A labor rate of $3.75 per hour
3.   When the machine in question is idle, labor costs are one half of those incurred when the machine is running
4.   Capacities: a 12 gross ton per hour incinerator, a 30 gross ton per hour baler, a 30 gross ton per hour shear, a 120 gross ton input per hour shredder (or about 92 gross ton per hour output), a 2.5 gross ton per hour (dust input) cyclone separator

Point 4 deserves further explanation. Note first that the capacities for the baler, shear, and shredder were chosen from the high end of the capacity range. These choices are significant for the following reasons: If investment per unit capacity and manpower per unit capacity (figure 6-3) are relatively constant—that is, independent of capacity—then plant size will not affect the optimal quantities of scrap which are shredded, baled, and sheared. This then indicates that the optimum values (with respect to type of scrap processing) generated by the linear program will be insensitive to variations in plant size. It is clear from the regression analyses run on investment costs for the processing equipment, all of the form

$$C_k = a_k + b_k Q_k$$

with a_k being about 0.0, that economies of scale in scrap processing equipment are very small. While an extensive study of process equipment costs would almost certainly reveal that a_k was slightly greater than 0.0, implying some small economies of scale, we may reasonably assume for purposes of the present study that the economies of scale are insignificant. Figure 6-7[31] reveals that for the cases of the baler and shear (and even for the shredder) manpower per unit capacity is not a relatively constant function of capacity. The effect of these deviations can be understood by considering the following points:
1.   If the baling and shearing operations in the region under consideration are in the 25–35 gross ton per hour capacity range, then the optimum values are essentially insensitive to plant size
2.   In any event, the linear programming model presented can reasonably be expected to mimic the behavior of the regional scrap

---

[31] In order to obtain a continuous plot of manpower per gross ton per hour capacity versus capacity (figure 6-3) a linear relationship was assumed to hold between manpower and capacity even though in actual fact such a relationship does not exist (as previously stated). The purpose of figure 6-3 is to give some insight into the problem of determining whether the linear program solutions will be sensitive or insensitive to plant size.

market in the case where the great majority of balers and shears are operating at capacities of about 30 gross tons per hour[32]

3. Economies of scale would have to be quite significant (that is, a_k would have to be quite large) before the supply or the elasticity of supply of scrap, as predicted by the model, would change

The cyclone separator and incinerator data were not subject to the preceding analysis since all the cyclone separator data are based on cost estimates, and the incinerator data were generated by the power method from a single datum.

With these assumptions and qualifications, the following fixed plus semivariable process costs were used in the model:

1. Incineration: $2.80 per gross ton output
2. Baling: $2.82 per gross ton input or output
3. Shearing: $4.18 per gross ton input or output
4. Shredding: $5.24 per gross ton input; $6.85 per gross ton output
5. Dust collection (cyclone separator): $1.97 per gross ton of dust input

THE HULK PROCESSING MODEL

The final step is the assembly of the total processing model. Let x_k represent the number of hulks to be purchased from annulus k. Let c_k represent the cost of a hulk from auto dismantling plus the cost of transportation from annulus k to Philadelphia, and let b_k represent the availability of auto hulks in annulus k.

This information is incorporated in the process analysis model objective function of maximizing profits V, as

$$V = \ldots \sum_{k=1}^{p} \ldots - c_k x_k \ldots$$

with the inequalities

$$0 \leq x_k \leq b_k \qquad k = 1, 2, \ldots, p$$

acting as constraints for p annuli. This is the traditional linear version of the programming problem.

The remainder of the model is constructed from material balance, number balance, and constraint equations. All the equations are linear,

---

[32] Suppose, however, that either (a) this is not the case, or (b) the modeller's need for accuracy is extremely great, and requires the most nearly perfect results attainable. In this case a mixed integer linear program formulation may be used (the small number of processes would result in reasonable solution times on a large-scale digital computer). This would generate globally optimal solutions in spite of the problem of economies of scale. See N. J. Driebeek, *Applied Linear Programming* (Addison-Wesley, Reading, Mass., 1969), pp. 119–140.

and together form a complete mathematical description of the scrap processing system shown in the flow chart in figure 2-2. These equations constitute a mixed integer linear programming problem, since integer values of hulks are fed to a baler, shear, or shredder. But the number of auto hulks being fed is very large (on the order of hundreds of thousands). Thus, on the practical level, a fraction of a car can simply be rounded off to the nearest integer with no serious mathematical error.

Constraints built into the model include capacity constraints on the baler, the baler-shear, the open burning of hulks, the incineration of hulks, the shredder, and the particulates produced (from burning or shredding of hulks). The construction of the model is such that it is a trivial matter to add or delete constraints, and it is relatively simple even to add or delete processes. The model calculates, for any set of costs and constraints, the optimum operating levels for all equipment to produce maximum profits; the number of hulks (if any) to be purchased from each annulus; the number of hulks to be burned in the open; the number to be incinerated; the number left unburned; the number to be sheared; the number to be baled; the number to be shredded; the number of tons of the different types of scrap to be produced; the particulates produced; the energy and water used; and the actual profit in dollars per year.

The model mimics the behavior of the aggregate of scrap processors in a metropolitan area. It maximizes profits, subject to the prevailing technological, economic, and legal climates. If all the prices and costs are fixed, it calculates the optimum amount of scrap to be produced in each of several types of equipment, and the maximum radius from the processing center from which cars can be profitably purchased—thereby calculating the quantity of raw material supplied and the quantity of processed scrap to be supplied. By utilizing parametric programming, which is a method of sequentially varying one or more prices or costs over a series of runs, letting the other prices and costs remain constant, a series of runs can be made which furnishes a set of couplets, each consisting of a quantity supplied and a price offered. These, of course, are the points of a supply function.

The parametric variation of scrap prices can be seen as the driving force for the model. If scrap prices are initially set at some low level— low enough so that the model (processors) cannot make a profit—and then successively raised to average and high values, the model will initially buy no cars and make no scrap. As scrap prices increase, the model will begin to buy those hulks produced nearby. As prices rise even further, the model, trying constantly to produce more and more profits, will buy cars farther and farther from the location of the hypothetical central processor. Thus scrap supply will increase and the number of abandoned automobiles decrease as scrap prices increase.

Moreover, transportation costs in the model include both (a) those of hulk shipment and (b) those of shipment from the processor to the steel company. In the case of hulk shipment, the price of driving a truckload of hulks a certain number of miles tends to be a constant, essentially independent of the number of hulks on the truck. As a result, the model always has trucks carry as many hulks as the modeller allows. From this derives the conclusion, to be amplified in the next chapter, that the number of hulks carried per truckload affects the quantity of processed scrap supplied at any specified scrap price. And, as a result, the elasticity of supply varies with the number of hulks carried per truck.

In the case of the processed scrap shipping cost, it may be set to any level desired by the modeller. It affects the profitability of making the processed scrap; therefore it affects the supply. Processed scrap shipping costs, which will vary with the distance from the processor to the steel mill, were arbitrarily set at $2 per gross ton. This number was based on conversations with the scrap processors interviewed.

This completes the discussion of the structure of the hulk processing model.[33] It includes all those considerations which are of interest: the population density distribution of the region, the availability of de-registered automobiles throughout the region, hulk transportation costs, fixed and semivariable processing costs (with all their implied pertinent variables), variable processing costs, solid residuals generation, air-borne particulate residuals generation, noxious gas formation, and trans-portation of the processed scrap. The model is so constructed that the values of any or all of the relevant independent variables may be readily changed, and new process options easily added. Thus, its con-struction facilitates experimenting with either historical information or hypothetical cases of interest to the user.

Analyses conducted with the model are discussed in chapter 7. The analyses made always yielded results which were plausible in their own right or corroborated (and elucidated) some previous investigator's re-sults. As is well known (see de Neufville and Stafford[34]), such models are difficult, if not impossible, to verify completely. The best test of the model will be in continued experimenting over a wide range of feasible solution space and checking whether the results are plausible. The second most reliable method of model verification is an ever-critical examina-

---

[33] The mathematics of the model are simple but too lengthy to be enclosed here. They are given in detail in an unpublished doctoral dissertation, "A Regional Model of the Automobile Scrap Processing Sector of the Economy," by J. W. Sawyer, University of Pennsylvania, 1973; available from University Microfilms, Ann Arbor, Michigan.

[34] Richard de Neufville and Joseph H. Stafford, *Systems Analysis for Engineers and Managers* (McGraw-Hill, 1971).

tion of the equations involved and their coefficients. Within the limits of the research carried out, the coefficients seem reasonably correct. Unfortunately, however, the processes studied have never received the amount of attention that is routinely devoted to far less common technologies. It is probably safe to say that the quantitative characteristics of the most exotic transistor have been established far more precisely than those of the most common types of steel scrap processing equipment. Such a situation offers a serious challenge to the modeller. The first models must be constructed with care, but prolonged study of each coefficient is neither possible nor fruitful.

Even deciding which coefficients should receive the most attention is not a simple problem.[35] Nonetheless, the model makes explicit what data are needed. The current interest in environmental problems will help to ensure that the necessary data will become available, as can be recognized from the efforts now underway by the Environmental Protection Agency. Verifying the model, then, is seen as an evolutionary process. Its use will prompt new research which, in turn, will prompt model revision.

[35] See W. O. Spofford, Jr., and H. A. Thomas, Jr., "A Least Cost Evaluation of Disposal Systems for Low Level Liquid Radioactive Wastes: Simplified Deterministic Model," *Transport of Radionuclides in Fresh Water Systems*, U.S. Atomic Energy Commission, Division of Technical Information, TID-7664, July 1963.

7

Analysis and Synthesis

The preceding chapters have described the steel scrap industry: the raw material, the processes used, the products made, the quality problems associated with the output of processed steel scrap, and a model of the production of automobile-derived steel scrap. This chapter discusses those particular features of the industry, whether explored by mathematical models or by qualitative analysis, which are of greatest interest to persons concerned with environmental quality and natural resources management.

ELASTICITY OF SUPPLY OF STEEL SCRAP DERIVED FROM OBSOLETE AUTOMOBILES

The concept of supply includes three subcategories:[1] the very short-run (or market period) supply function, the short-run supply function, and the long-run supply function. Elasticity of supply is defined as the percentage change in quantity supplied resulting from a 1 percent change in price [mathematically this is stated as being $(\Delta Q/Q)/(\Delta P/P)$, where Q represents quantity supplied and P represents price and $\Delta P/P = 1\%$]. In the very short run, the quantity of a good supplied is fixed and the elasticity of supply is near zero. For example, a person who desires to buy a specific suit from a specific store might find that once an initial suit is purchased, he cannot buy an identical suit regardless of the price he offers. However, in the short run (a few weeks in our example) the elasticity might be significantly greater than zero because the store may be able to obtain a new shipment of the required suits. Finally, the elasticity of supply in the long run will be even greater, since in the

---

[1] See J. M. Henderson and R. E. Quandt, *Microeconomic Theory: A Mathematical Approach* (McGraw-Hill, 1971), pp. 108–111.

long run the store not only can obtain several shipments of the desired suits, but also can modify its merchandising patterns so that the specific suit becomes a feature item. This discussion points to two important facts: (a) discussions of supply must specify the time period under consideration; (b) as the time period increases so also does the elasticity of supply.

Estimates of the supply of steel scrap in the literature to date have been of two types, econometric and analytic. The econometric studies made on steel scrap, while offering insight into the workings of the national scrap market, fail to explicate the effect of structural variables[2] on supply in the regional marketplace. Therefore, they cannot confidently be used to discuss the supply of scrap in a time period other than that for which the statistical analysis was made.

The supply of ferrous scrap and measurement of the elasticity of supply have been studied from an econometric standpoint by a series of workers. According to Plater-Zyberk, the domestic scrap industry has not to date (1971) permitted any in-depth analysis of scrap sources and their recovery practices. He found this to be the case, also, among local scrap dealers. Accordingly, he feels that the data available on scrap supply are of poor quality and of no use in formulating a supply equation for use in a dynamic market model.[3]

Adams, by using econometric techniques, attempted to estimate the national supply function of ferrous scrap. His analysis was on a monthly time series of data for the period 1963–1971, so that his supply equations would normally be considered to be short run (1–2 years). He derived supply equations for both No. 2 Bundles and No. 1 Heavy Melting, the latter being chosen as a surrogate variable for shredded scrap.[4] While he did not estimate elasticity, calculations with his data indicate U.S. elasticities of supply of shredded scrap of about ten (at average Philadelphia scrap prices of $31.50 per gross ton for No. 1 Heavy Melting). The difficulties with his analysis will be discussed below.

Adams also made some econometric studies of the supply and demand

[2] Examples of structural variables are the number of cars shipped per truckload, the population density distribution, the cost of flattening a car, the rate of deregistration of automobiles, and all the other independent variables in the model.

[3] R. Plater-Zyberk, "The Economics of Ferrous Scrap Recycling," unpublished Ph.D. thesis, Drexel University, Philadelphia, Pa., 1972, pp. 112, 133.

[4] This is acceptable, even if not exactly true, on the demand side. On the supply side, however, it would seem to be totally unacceptable. The supply function for No. 2 Shredded Scrap should be more closely related to the supply function for No. 2 Bundles (since they are both made from the same raw materials) than to the supply function for No. 1 Heavy Melting. Thus the use of elasticities for shredded scrap derived from Adams' equations for No. 1 Heavy Melting appears open to serious question.

for No. 2 Bundles. While he proposes a number of equations, and does not calculate elasticities of supply, his apparently best equation choice gives relationships which indicate an elasticity of supply (1971) of about eight. Over a period of years the elasticity of supply seems to be in the range of five to ten.[5]

Johnson[6] also estimated the elasticity of supply of ferrous scrap. The supply equation he developed related the quantity of No. 2 Bundles to annual scrappage of cars and trucks and the annual average price of No. 2 Bundles. He found the short-term elasticity of supply of bundled ferrous scrap to be very small, in the 0.01–0.02 range. This indicates that the supply of bundled ferrous scrap is extremely inelastic. Johnson attributes this result to poor data or the increased role of shredded scrap, which is not included in No. 2 Bundle data. He thinks there should be some response of supply to price although it does not appear empirically.[7] Johnson utilized data from the late 1950s to the middle 1960s, and does not state whether he has estimated a very short run, a short-run, or a long-run supply equation. However, in the latter part of his paper, he performs calculations which imply that he considered it a short-term supply function.

The Bureau of Mines has found the short-run elasticity of supply for No. 2 Bundles to be about one.[8] That study utilized quarterly data from January 1963 to March 1965. The Bureau of Mines researchers developed a supply function that relates the quantity of No. 2 Bundles supplied to the real price[9] of No. 2 Bundles in the preceding time period. This study assumed away the well-known identification problem in econometric analyses, however, thereby seriously reducing the credibility of the results.

There are two major problems with the preceding diverse estimates. First, the econometric analyses give no insight into the effect the variables or processes present in the scrap-producing sequence have on

---

[5] Later in this chapter it is argued that the elasticity of supply of No. 2 Bundles is indeed five to ten, and that the demand for highly contaminated scrap, such as No. 2 Bundles, is inelastic. A calculated arc elasticity of demand for No. 2 Bundles from Adams' work is about 0.1, thereby supporting the argument. It is noteworthy that Adams' equation formulation for the demand for No. 2 Bundles includes only the production rate of steel in open hearth and electric arc furnaces, rather than total steel production.

[6] See William R. Johnson, "The Supply and Demand for Scrapped Automobiles," *Western Economic Journal*, vol. IX (1971), pp. 441–443.

[7] *Ibid.*, p. 442.

[8] See U.S. Department of the Interior, Bureau of Mines, *Automobile Disposal, A National Problem*, 1967, pp. 69–70.

[9] Real price is defined as average monthly price of No. 2 Bundles divided by the GNP implied price deflator which is chosen as a representative of the general cost trend.

the elasticities calculated. The second is that econometric approaches[10] used by previous researchers cannot easily handle the effects of technological changes which were significant for the periods under consideration. For instance, after 1963 (see figure 7-1), use of the basic oxygen

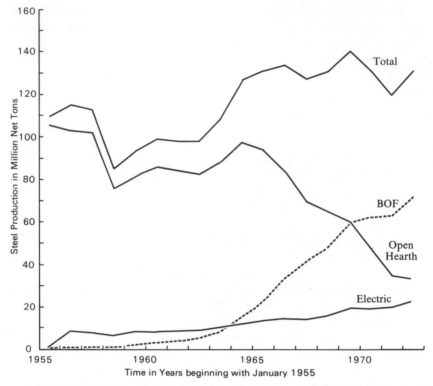

FIGURE 7-1. Steel production by various techniques. Data from AISI yearbook for 1971.

furnace (BOF) increased substantially, while use of the open hearth furnace decreased.[11] Other recent technological changes are the flattening of auto hulks before shipment and the shift from baling to shredding as the primary method of processing hulks.

[10] Concerning econometric analysis, it should be noted that there are certain mathematical difficulties in statistically estimating two curves (supply and demand) from one set of data (price and quantity). See especially R. L. Adams, "An Economic Analysis of the Junk Automobile Problem," unpublished Ph.D. dissertation, Department of Economics, University of Illinois, 1972; and Richard de Neufville and Joseph H. Stafford, *Systems Analysis for Engineers and Managers* (McGraw-Hill, 1971), pp. 294–295.

[11] Open hearth furnace steel production can utilize far more scrap than BOF steel production.

In the analytical approach, the supply of raw feed for scrap processes (that is, obsolete automobiles) is taken to be the amount of a given type of manufactured good that was produced τ years before, τ being the average lifetime of the manufactured good under examination. This approach has been extensively utilized by such students of the scrap problem as Battelle.[12] The history of the analytic approach is reviewed, and the concept is extensively criticized by Gordon et al.[13] They point out that the problem with this approach is fundamental. To treat the supply of something as independent of the cost is to abandon the economists' traditional concept of supply (that is, supply as a function of price) and to cause it to lose its explanatory power.

In this study, the approach has been to use the analytical approach to determine what has been dubbed "availability." Clearly, when an automobile is deregistered, it becomes available—at least potentially— as raw material for the scrap processor. If the price offered for obsolete automobiles is sufficiently high to bring the available automobiles into the scrap market, they become part of the supply as traditionally defined by the economist.

Discussions of supply of processed scrap are particularly difficult compared with other commodities, regardless of methodology. For, as pointed out by Vogely[14] and Gordon et al.,[15] the physical availability of raw obsolete scrap is excessive, in the sense that there is unused scrap lying about, in periods of low price. Should the price of scrap be increased by some increment, Δ, there will be some increase in supply up to some price at which all the physically available scrap is consumed. While the elasticity of supply of scrap may have been (relatively) constant up to that time, it will then drop instantly to zero.[16] That is, there

[12] See Battelle Memorial Institute, *A Survey and Analysis of the Supply and Availability of Obsolete Iron and Steel Scrap*, Report to the Business and Defense Services Administration, Department of Commerce, Columbus, Ohio, 1957.

[13] See Richard L. Gordon, Wilfrid A. Lambo, and George H. K. Schenck, *Effective Systems of Scrap Utilization: Copper, Aluminum, and Nickel*, Report to the U.S. Department of the Interior, Bureau of Mines, The Pennsylvania State University, University Park, Pa. (undated but probably published in 1972).

[14] See William A. Vogely, "The Economic Factors of Mineral Waste Utilization," *Proceedings of the Symposium: Mineral Waste Utilization*, sponsored by the U.S. Bureau of Mines and IIT Research Institute, Chicago, 1968.

[15] Gordon et al., *Effective Systems*.

[16] This will be true, of course, only if increases in scrap metal prices cannot affect scrappage rates. For post-consumer scrap in general, and for obsolete automobiles in particular, this is probably a good assumption, at least for the normal variations in scrap process. It would be surprising if the variation in deregistration rates with scrap metal costs were significantly greater than zero.

Nevertheless, the general problem of the variation in scrappage rates with scrap prices is a matter of interest to the environmental student. Should the reader wish to pursue this problem further, a thorough and thoughtful analysis of the research to date is given in Richard L. Gordon et al., *Effective Systems*.

is a (potential) discontinuity in the short-term (1–3 years) steel scrap supply curve.

This brief discussion of the work done to date on ferrous scrap supply serves to introduce our calculation of supply of ferrous scrap from obsolete autos. First, the supply functions are calculated under the assumptions that there is a surplus of physically available scrap. That is, all calculations refer to that portion of the function below the kink (or discontinuity) in the raw scrap supply curve. Thus, they would be inapplicable in a situation in which governmental economic policy or technological change moved the demand curve so that the quantity demanded was near the kink in the supply curve. Second, the supply curves calculated herein are of the short-term class, that is, for one to two, perhaps slightly more, years.[17] To assume that they would apply for longer periods than this would be to assume a cessation of new construction in the scrap industry, which is unlikely. Third, the supply curves calculated are for a specific geographic region (Philadelphia) and a specific set of materials costs, production costs, and product prices, and they assume a $3.75 per hour wage rate. Fourth, it was assumed that the price paid for hulks is $10, and is independent of the price paid for processed scrap. Fifth, the model developed here is static, and applies at market equilibrium. Its results will of necessity be less than perfect in a period of technological transition. The supply functions calculated here, then, are for an industry of an assumed structure, a structure modeled after that of the scrap industry in the Philadelphia area.[18] Nonetheless, the results can be used, along with verbal analysis, to cast light on the nature of postconsumer scrap supply as well as the steel scrap market in general.

Using the hulk processing models discussed above, the supplies of No. 2 Bundles and shredded scrap were calculated for the Philadelphia area. It was assumed in the calculation that the present air pollution regulations are enforced[19] and that the shredder in Philadelphia (there is currently only one shredder) has a capacity of 750 cars per day, or 187,500 cars per operational year (250 days). Moreover, it was assumed that there was little demand for sheared scrap or burned scrap of any

---

[17] A short enough period of time that new processing capacity cannot be installed.

[18] The model is quite general. As better data become available on raw material costs, operating costs, transportation costs, and population distribution, or if someone wants to model a different region, these data should be used in the model to give a better idea of how the supply of scrap varies with price.

[19] The maximum allowable discharge rate for particulates in Philadelphia is 40 parts per hundred or 83,200 pounds of particulates per year; see City of Philadelphia, Air Management Regulation V of the Air Pollution Control Board (1971).

sort (an unrealistic assumption that was made to simplify the presentation of data—the supply and the elasticity of supply could be calculated for any and all combinations of processes).[20] The supply data were calculated for a series of assumptions about the number of flattened cars which would be shipped per truckload if flattening were employed, even though a series of counts of hulks per truck indicated the usual value to be about twenty.

The average price of shredded scrap in the Philadelphia area was about $31.50 per gross ton for the period January 1966 through December 1971. These prices are at the steel company's location, and the scrap processor pays the cost of transportation. (See appendix A.) At this price the calculated supply of shredded scrap is about 143,800 gross tons per year, or about 187,500 auto hulks per year (this is constrained by the capacity of the shredder).[21] The average price of No. 2 Bundles in the Philadelphia area was about $21.50 per gross ton (1966 through 1971), and at this price the calculated supply of No. 2 Bundles is on the order of 50,000 gross tons (but varying greatly with the number of flattened cars shipped per truck), or about 50,000 auto hulks. This is a total of about 237,500 auto hulks per year, or about 20,000 auto hulks per month. Increasing the price by only $1 per ton (to $32.50 for shredded scrap and $22.50 for No. 2 Bundles) increases the quantity supplied to about 430,000 hulks per year, or about 35,000 hulks per month. These numbers are good approximations to Plater-Zyberk's estimate (which he considered highly tentative) of 25–35,000 hulks per month, a figure which he obtained by interviewing brokers in the Philadelphia area. Plater-Zyberk did not estimate the variation in supply with price.[22]

If the price is raised another dollar per ton, there is sufficient economic incentive to use all the deregistered cars becoming available within a 100-mile radius of Philadelphia (New York City excepted), which is one of the limits of the model with its present coefficients.

Summary results in the form of calculated price elasticities of supply and gross profits (before taxes) of the scrap industry in the Philadelphia

[20] To calculate the supplies and the elasticities without these restrictive assumptions requires more information than is currently available on the capacities of the various processes for the Philadelphia region.

[21] At the point at which shredder capacity is fully utilized, of course, the elasticity of supply of shredded scrap becomes zero. The overall study reveals that shredding is significantly more profitable than either baling or shearing. Thus the model suggests that shredding capacity in Philadelphia will expand rapidly to remove this constraint. And indeed, this seems to be the case, since two dealers indicated during interview trips that they were going to buy shredders.

[22] Plater-Zyberk, "The Economics of Ferrous Scrap."

TABLE 7-1.   Elasticity of Supply[a] for Steel Scrap in Philadelphia and
Magnitude of Auto Scrap Market

Number of cars per truck if not flattened	Number of cars per truck if flattened	Elasticity of supply for auto hulks	Elasticity of supply for No. 2 Bundles[b]	Elasticity of supply for No. 2 Bundles if baler capacity is exceeded by demand	Elasticity of supply for shredded scrap	Elasticity of supply for shredded scrap if demand exceeds shredder capacity	To va͏l of s͏o out i͏n milli͏o doll
6	Not applicable	4	4	0	6	0	0.4
6	20	4	16	0	20	0	1.0
6	25	5	20	0	25	0	1.3
6	30	10	24	0	31	0	1.5
6	35	15	28	0	36	0	1.6
6	40	20	32	0	41	0	1.7

[a] The significance of elasticity of supply figures can be simply expressed as follows: if the offer price of a good is increased by 1 percent, the percentage increase in its supply equals its elasticity. example, in the early 1960s before flattening technology was available (row 1 of the table), an incre of 1 percent in the price of No. 2 Bundles would have resulted in an increase of 4 percent in quantity supplied.

[b] As indicated in appendix A to chapter 7, the average price in Philadelphia of No. 2 Bundles the period January 1966 through December 1971 was about $21.50 per gross ton; for No. 1 He Melting, which has a price similar to that of shredded scrap, it was $31.50 per gross ton. To obt the arc elasticities reported in this table, the model was started with an initial price of $15 per gross for No. 2 Bundles and $25 per gross ton for shredded scrap. Then a series of runs was made, creasing the price of each of the two types of scrap $0.25 per gross ton for each of the two types scrap until all the cars within a 100-mile radius of Philadelphia were consumed. In all cases, signific quantities of scrap were not processed until the price had risen to $18–19 per gross ton (for No Bundles) and $28–29 per gross ton (for shredded scrap). In all cases except one (the nonflattened case), all the deregistered automobiles becoming available were being consumed by the time scr prices had increased to $20–24 per gross ton for No. 2 Bundles and $30–34 per gross ton for shredd scrap. Thus the arc elasticities reported are for the price of about $20–24 per gross ton for No. Bundles and $30–34 per gross ton for shredded scrap.

area are given in table 7-1.[23] The only elasticity values which approximate those estimated from Adams' econometric studies (for No. 2 Bundles) are associated with cars which are not flattened. In this special case, which approximated the real situation in the late 1960s that

[23] In calculating the elasticities, some difficulties were encountered because of the nature of the computer formulation. Elasticity is, by definition, a derivative function. That is

$$\eta = \frac{P}{Q}\left(\frac{\partial Q}{\partial P}\right)$$

where η represents price elasticity of supply, P represents price, and Q represents quantity supplied. Taking a derivative numerically is, of course, best accomplished by using very small increments. Unfortunately, in a model of the type made, the price of taking very small increments is a great increase in the number of rows, hence a great increase in solution time and cost. Thus, the price increment chosen was $0.25, which is comparatively large. As a result, there are a large number of discontinuities in the supply versus price curve, making excellent supplied the data for Adams' econometric studies, the calculated elasticity values are reasonably close to the econometric results (aggregated for the nation).

The method by which auto hulks are being shipped is changing rapidly. Traditionally hulks have been hauled unflattened from auto wrecking yards on flatbed trucks. Adams,[24] citing a Bureau of Mines survey of shredded scrap producers, says that in 1969, 60 percent of auto hulks were unflattened. These were shipped to the shredders on trucks carrying five to eight hulks per load. In contrast, the flattened hulks averaged twelve to twenty-five per load. Shredders who were not already receiving all their hulks in flattened condition indicated that they expected the number of flattened hulks to increase significantly. Combining this information with that from table 7-1 strongly suggests that the long-term price elasticity of supply of steel scrap may be expected to increase somewhat over the next few years. If it is currently about five (up to the price at which demand exceeds shredder capacity, at which elasticity becomes zero), the value might be expected to increase to ten, or perhaps slightly more.

It seems highly improbable that it will ever get as high as 20–40 with present technology. First, it cannot reasonably be expected that many trucks will carry more than twenty cars. Most will carry six to twenty cars. Second, it seems improbable that a flattening cost of $4.15 per car (the value used here) will prevail universally. This figure assumes that flatteners will be used about 50 percent of the time, perhaps a high estimate. It would seem to be the case that flatteners, even portable flatteners, will be used at a small fraction of their capacity, except for those few instances in which they are located in dismantling yards where there is a large volume of business. Thus, a flattening cost of $5 or even

---

approximation to $\partial Q/\partial P$ effectively impossible to obtain. In addition, further complications were introduced by the fact that there is a constraint on the size of the shredder, which comes into play at relatively low costs, and a total constraint in the number of available hulks because the region considered was arbitrarily limited to that geographical region lying within a 100-mile radius of Philadelphia. This latter constraint resulted in a relatively narrow price spread between the initial production of baled scrap and a production level of baled scrap which reached the limit of the available cars for the region.

With these problems in mind, problems which are well known to economists, the best solution was to calculate arc elasticities of supply. [See G. J. Stigler, *The Theory of Price*, 3rd ed. (Macmillan, 1966), pp. 331, 332.] This was done by (a) calculating the best $\Delta Q/\Delta P$ value possible under the circumstances, (b) plotting the calculated value of η as a function of the number of cars being transported by the flattener, and drawing smooth lines through the calculated points. The values (of arc elasticity of supply) in table 7-1 were taken from the smoothed curves.

[24] R. L. Adams, "Economic Analysis," chapter IV.

$6 per car might be more realistic. This would have a twofold effect. It would directly decrease the price elasticity of supply of the flattened auto hulks, and it would also shift to a greater distance from the scrap processor the point at which it would have been more economical to ship flattened than unflattened hulks. Thus, the price elasticities of supply would be well below the (maximum) values reported in table 7-1.[25]

Consideration of the various factors built into the model makes it relatively easy to see how the calculated elasticities can be quite high compared with what we might think intuitively. Assume that the price of processed scrap is such that all the cars are being processed that are deregistered within a 50-mile radius of Philadelphia (and none outside this radius). This implies a price for shredded scrap of about $31.50 per gross ton. Now suppose the price of scrap is increased 1 percent, to $31.82. With all other costs remaining constant, the increase in supply will simply be the additional transportation that can be paid for with this $0.32 increase in processed scrap price. At about 50 miles, from the transportation cost equation developed by Adams, the marginal cost per mile additional shipment for trucks carrying twenty hulks is about $0.04 per mile, so that a $0.32 increase in price will increase the distance of profitable shipment about 8 miles. This implies an enormous increase in the number of available hulks. The area of an annulus whose inner radius is 50 miles and whose outer radius is 58 miles is π $(58^2 - 50^2)$, or about 2700 square miles. At a distance of 50 miles from the city, population densities are of the order of magnitude of 480 per square mile. If 0.033 cars per person per year are deregistered, this implies an increase in the number of available hulks per year of $0.033 \times 200 \times 2700$, or about 42,000 hulks. The availability of hulks at $31.50 per gross ton for shredded scrap within a 50-mile radius of the city is about 187,500—or about 140,000 gross tons of shredded scrap (since only about 75 percent of the weight of each hulk is converted to salable shredded scrap). This admittedly rough calculation, then, suggests a percentage increase in supply of about $100 \times (42,000 \times 0.75/140,000)$, or about 20 percent, for a 1 percent increase in the offering price for processed scrap. Thus the explanation for the elasticities of supply of 20–40, as predicted by the model, can be readily understood with the aid of a simple calculation.[26]

How good are the estimates of elasticity given by the model and

[25] We have not quantitatively explored the effect of the ideas discussed here because of the limitation of time. The amount of effort required to describe fully the system of transporting auto hulks to Philadelphia would not seem to justify the marginal gain in insight into the price elasticity of steel scrap supply.

[26] The calculations in this paragraph are not intended to be exact. Rather, using rough estimates, the intention is to simply elucidate the high elasticity values obtained by the vastly greater, hence more precise, calculations using the full linear programming model.

what are the weakest links in the chain of reasoning leading to the results obtained? As already suggested, the higher elasticity values given are unrealistic, based on the problems involved in the assumptions concerning transportation—both flattening costs and the number of hulks shipped per truck. Another problem is that the price of hulks has been assumed to be a constant over time. It is true that this was a good approximation to the real behavior of the scrap market in the Philadelphia region throughout the study. But the interviews with scrap dealers were all held within the course of a year to a year and a half, and over that time the price of scrap was relatively constant. It is basically not realistic to suggest that there is no relationship between processed scrap prices and hulk prices. Rather, when processed scrap prices are very low, hulk prices are also low, while when processed scrap prices are very high, hulk prices tend to be higher than average.[27] Were data relating hulk prices to processed scrap prices available, their incorporation in the model used in this study would be straightforward. But such data are not available, and are relatively difficult to obtain except by repeated interviews with scrap processors over several years. The time required would depend on the time required for scrap prices to go through a couple of their cycles (see figure 7-11 in the appendix to this chapter). In the absence of these data, there was little choice but to assume a constant value for hulks.

The effect of the hulk price assumption on elasticity figures is not clear. If hulk prices do indeed rise as scrap prices rise, elasticities of supply will be lower than estimated here. The quantitative extent of this overestimation of elasticities is difficult to ascertain. Nonetheless, the presence of the problematical assumption is yet a second reason to suspect that short-run elasticities of supply cannot reasonably be expected to be higher than, say, five to ten, and indeed may not be as high as that.

A third and fourth consideration also lead us to be wary of the very high elasticity figures generated by the scrap processing model. There is the possibility that a sustained period of high demand—resulting in high price—could conceivably result in the elimination of all the available deregistered automobiles in the region. At this point one of the key assumptions on which the model is based would be violated, and the elasticity of supply would become zero. Finally, while 0.033 automobiles per person per year may be deregistered, that is no assurance that they all become available to the scrap market. A close examination of the explicit assumptions in the model suggests that the elasticity of supply of

---

[27] This phenomenon is well known to scrap processors. They think in terms of what they call the "spread," that is, the difference between what they pay for raw scrap and what they get paid for processed scrap. And the "spread," according to many dealers, has a tendency to remain fairly constant.

steel scrap may not be as high as the model implies. Nonetheless, despite all the caveats, it is clear that the supply of obsolete or post-consumer steel scrap is elastic.

Another consideration suggests that, under special circumstances, the elasticity of supply may be higher than the model suggests. It is common knowledge that in the economic boom of 1973, industry was operating at 90–95 percent of capacity. But the scrap industry, as the processors now run their operations, is operating at about 40 percent of capacity. Thus, should scrap prices rise (and they have been rising dramatically since late 1972) and stay high (which in view of the long-term history of scrap prices seems unlikely—see appendix A), there would be a large incentive for scrap processors to change their mode of operation, and expand to 80–90 percent of the true capacity of the industry. This possibility, seldom broached, arises from the fact that scrap processors operate their equipment 8–10 hours per day, and usually 5 days per week. Most continuous process industries operate 168 hours per week except in the case of shutdown for repairs or preventive maintenance. Assuming a conservative figure of 6 hours preventive maintenance per day, the average shredder, which now operates about 50 hours per week, could operate about 130 hours per week.

If this is the case, then it may be asked why, as scrap prices rise rapidly, as they have since the fall of 1972, scrap processors do not dramatically expand their output? Two explanations seem plausible. First, there would undoubtedly be significant costs involved in switching from a one-shift operation to a four-shift operation. While these costs could easily be justified if scrap prices rose to high levels and stayed at high levels, the past history of the market strongly suggests that this will not be the case (barring some structural change in the international scrap market similar to that now suggested by some economists as having occurred in the world food market). Thus, a canny scrap processor would not take the step of expanding to a four-shift operation until he had greater reason to believe than has yet been offered that scrap prices were leveling out at an equilibrium level well above that previously established. Nonetheless, the fact remains that over the short term (1–2 years) scrap processing capacity could be expanded on the order of 100–150 percent with no new plant construction, and at relatively low cost. Thus, the present operating practices of the scrap processor offer assurance that a significant and permanent increase in the price of scrap could certainly result in dramatic increases in the supply of processed scrap (up to the level of availability of deregistered automobiles).

A second consideration that would result in elasticities of supply being higher than either the model or intuition would suggest is the commodity nature of the steel scrap market. While some commodity markets are stabilized by the mechanism of a futures market, the steel scrap market is not. As a result, the severe price fluctuations for scrap are an open invitation for speculation by dealers. Thus, among many dealers there is a pronounced tendency to build inventory during periods of low prices, and deplete inventory with the onset of high scrap prices. Such a practice will of course tend to increase scrap supply with increasing price more rapidly than would otherwise be the case. This practice of speculation, while common among dealers, is far from universal. Many dealers instead emphasize the continued flow of material and inventory minimization, even in times of relatively depressed scrap prices.

FURTHER COMMENTS ON SUPPLY

The preceding discussion, after considering a mathematical model of the scrap processing industry for a typical large industrial city, and many of the problems involved in capturing the complexity of the steel scrap industry in such a model, leads inexorably to the conclusion that the supply of scrap is elastic. This being the case, what is the explanation for the erratic nature of steel scrap prices (see figure 7-11)?

A number of relevant points can be made. First, the supply of steel scrap is elastic only up to the limit of equipment capacity (and raw material availability). When demand exceeds equipment capacity for a given type of steel scrap, there will be *no* relationship between price and quantity supplied, that is, there will be total inelasticity. Thus the supply function is highly elastic for small price differentials, then completely inelastic. It is obvious that such a situation would result in the dramatic price fluctuations so characteristic of steel scrap. There is good reason to believe that in the case of shredded scrap such a situation obtains. There is enormous shredder capacity in the United States, but this does not necessarily imply that there is adequate shredder capacity, since both the supply and the demand for steel scrap are highly regional in nature. In Philadelphia, for example, something on the order of two to three times as much shredder capacity could be used as is currently available. Moreover, an examination of shredded scrap production data for the United States reveals that since January 1970, when monthly data for both exports and imports began to be collected by the U.S. Bureau of Mines, shredded scrap production has increased relentlessly, being only modestly swerved from its normal path by shredded scrap price changes. In early 1970, total shredded scrap production was about 150,000 net tons per month. By early 1973, total shredded scrap production was about 300,000 net tons per month. By the middle of 1973, production was up to 350,000 net tons per month. This amounts to a 20–25 percent per year growth rate in shredded scrap production, a growth rate relatively unaffected by scrap prices, and showing no signs of slowing down. (See figures 7-2 and 7-3). Surely this must be taken as an indication

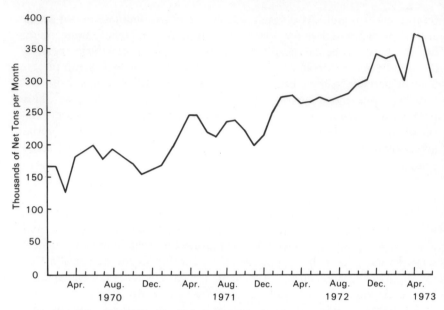

FIGURE 7-2.   Quantity supplied, both domestic and exported, of shredded scrap, expressed as a 3-month running average in thousands of net tons per month.

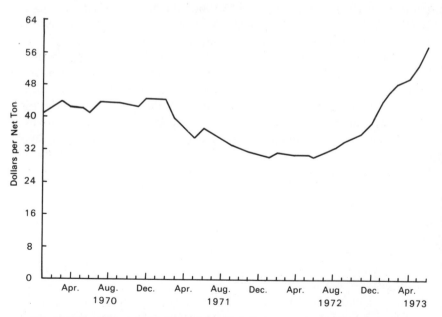

FIGURE 7-3.   Price of shredded scrap, in dollars per net ton. Data from declared values of export shredded scrap at dockside; 3-month running average.

that, in recent years, the scrap industry has had insufficient shredder capacity, and therefore should have behaved as if the short-term supply were inelastic. And indeed the calculated elasticities of supply are zero if capacity is insufficient.

What of bundled scrap? Slowly but surely the baler has been technologically superseded by the shredder. Not only is the demand for shredded scrap greater (presumably because of its quality), but, given the historically prevailing differences in price between shredded scrap and bundled scrap, shredding is much more profitable to the scrap dealer than baling. Thus, there is an excess of baling (and shearing) capacity. When scrap prices are normal, shredder-based scrap operations can more effectively compete for the raw material, that is, auto hulks. Baler-based processors gradually shut down. Then, when scrap prices rise, the shredder cannot meet the demand, and the baler-based processor has his evanescent day in the sun. If his equipment is still running, or if he can easily start it up, he can make a large profit. If he has previously shut down his baler, and cannot reactivate it with little effort, he has a gambler's choice. He can hope for a long period of high scrap prices, and reactivate his baling operations, or he can count on prices being only temporarily high, and make an educated guess that he will not make a sufficient profit in the short time prices will remain high to pay for the reactivation of his equipment. If this somewhat dismal view of the bundled scrap market is valid, it would be reflected in a gradual diminution in the output of baled scrap. Such indeed has been the case. In 1963, bundled scrap production was on the order of 550 thousand net tons per month; in 1966, 500; in 1969, 350; in 1973, 300 (in spite of extraordinarily high prices for bundled scrap in 1973). (See figure 7-4; for associated price data see figure 7-11.)

In short, technological transition in the scrap industry is the order of the day. Shredding first appeared in the early to mid-1960s. By 1975 to 1980, shredders may be expected to dominate the automobile-derived scrap portion of the scrap steel industry.

A quest for the explanation for variations in scrap prices, given the hypothesis that the automobile-derived steel scrap supply is elastic, reveals yet another facet of the scrap problem besides technological transition and capacity constraints. Referring to the discussion types of steel scrap in chapter 1, we can now see the significance of the fact that obsolete scrap is only about 40 percent by weight of total purchased scrap, and that automobile-derived scrap is only about 50–60 percent of all obsolete scrap. In this study, two types of automobile-derived obsolete scrap have been considered—shredded and bundled. The price of shredded scrap is essentially equal to that of No. 1 scrap in general (for evidence, see section 2, appendix A). But, while (currently) some

0.3 million short tons of shredded scrap are sold per month, some 2.5–3.0 million short tons of No. 1 scrap are sold per month. Thus, it is only reasonable to infer that the price of shredded scrap is completely dominated by the demand and supply for No. 1 (in general) rather than the demand and supply for shredded scrap. That is, No. 1 and shredded, from the viewpoint of ferrous materials manufacturing, are near-perfect substitutes.

It would be astonishing if the price elasticity of shredded scrap supply (which is high) was similar to the price elasticity of supplies of No. 1, which is almost certain to be inelastic, since the source of No. 1 is nearly all prompt scrap, the supply of which must be effectively independent of offering price. That is, the amount of prompt scrap generated at a specific steel production rate is, for all practical purposes, technologically fixed. If this were the sole source of all No. 1 scrap, the supply curve would be completely inelastic in the short run. Since obsolete scrap plays a very minor role as a source of No. 1 (see chapter 1), we can reason that the supply of No. 1 is nearly inelastic with respect to price.

Adams, in attempting to calculate a supply function for shredded scrap, developed a function from which it can be inferred that the

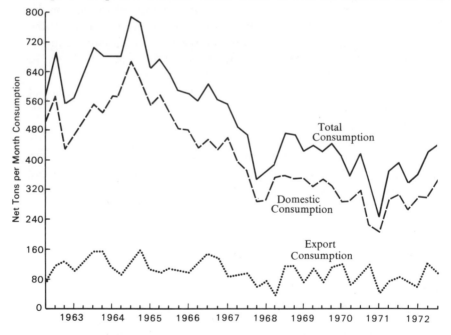

FIGURE 7-4. Total consumption, both domestic and abroad, of No. 2 bundles versus time. Data from *Mineral Industries Surveys*, U.S. Bureau of Mines (data expressed as quarterly averages).

elasticity of supply is five to ten. But he erroneously used No. 1 scrap as a proxy variable for shredded scrap. This is reasonable on the demand side, but not on the supply side, hence his calculations are of little value as far as shredded scrap is concerned. Moreover, another problem has eliminated the potential value of Adams' calculations as a predictor of the elasticity of supply of even No. 1 Heavy Melting. Adams used No. 1 Heavy Melting values (both prices and quantities) throughout his analysis, and his equations hypothesized that the quantity of No. 1 Heavy Melting demanded was directly proportional to steel production. But he failed to include in his formulation of the supply equation the obvious relationship between No. 1 Heavy Melting supply and steel production. As steel production increases, the supply of No. 1 Heavy Melting increases concomitantly. That is, the quantity supplied of No. 1 Heavy Melting increases in direct proportion to steel production. Adams' formulation of the problem failed to accommodate this fact. Thus, his results are not valid for shredded or No. 1 scrap.

In the case of bundled scrap, (a) which is not a substitute for No. 1 scrap and (b) for which production capacity is not limiting, the conclusions of Adams' econometric studies and the work reported here are in general agreement. Moreover, since equipment capacity is not limiting, it follows that the time pattern of No. 2 Bundle prices will be less erratic than that of No. 1 Heavy Melting prices. That this appears to be the case can be seen from figure 7-11.

The use of enormous amounts of prompt scrap has previously confounded an understanding of the supply of obsolete scrap. When prompt scrap represents some 60 percent of all purchased scrap, how could prompt scrap supply and demand fail to dominate the market's behavior?

Finally, then, it is concluded that the model presented here, in spite of all the caveats presented, gives a plausible starting point for thinking about the supply, and the elasticity of supply, of obsolete scrap. The supply of obsolete scrap, whether shredded, sheared, or baled, is indeed elastic, and the elasticity is about five to ten.

SIGNIFICANCE OF THE SUPPLY FUNCTION

The preceding discussion on supply serves as background information for discussing the larger problem of recycling. For a region of relatively high population density, on the order of 100 persons per square mile or more, the elasticity of supply at market equilibrium conditions is fairly high. As an initial approach to the problem of determining socially optimum recycling rates, those trained in economics would

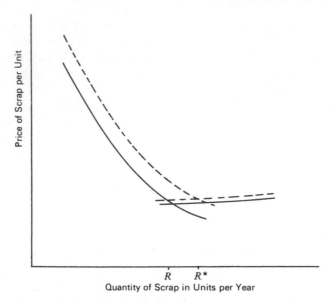

FIGURE 7-5.   A supply and demand diagram for one grade of steel scrap.
Dashed lines indicate comparable supply and demand functions when all social
costs are internalized. R designates recycling rate under current laws, R* designates
Pareto optimal recycling rate.

suggest that, given a free market system, economically optimum recycling rates will occur at the point where the supply function intersects
the demand function, with the proviso that all external costs are internalized in the market. This leads to the simple supply–demand diagram for one type of steel scrap shown in figure 7-5. The supply curve
is shown as a nearly horizontal line in accordance with the established
elasticity of supply at five to ten. The solid lines indicate the supply
and demand curves as now existing and the dotted lines indicate the
supply and demand curve in a situation where all external costs are internalized in the decision processes of the firms involved.

A great deal of the residuals production in the steelmaking process
arises from the production of iron in the blast furnace and the production
of the coke necessary for use in this furnace. The cost of reducing this
residuals production can reasonably be expected to be relatively high.[28]
By contrast, in the processing of post-consumer scrap, while significant
residuals are produced, the cost of reducing the discharges seems to be
low, as judged by the findings in this study (this is discussed further
below). Thus, if all external costs are internalized in the decision-making
processes of both steel production firms and scrap processing firms, it

[28] C. S. Russell and W. J. Vaughan, "A Linear Programming Model of Residuals
Management for Integrated Iron and Steel Production," to appear in *Journal of
Economics and Environmental Management*, vol. 1, no. 1.

can be reasonably expected that the demand for scrap at a given price might rise perceptibly (since it is competing with iron from blast furnaces) while the supply of scrap at a given price might decrease only slightly. This is expressed in figure 7-5 by the relative positions of the dotted and solid curves.

It has been repeatedly suggested throughout this monograph that scrap quality is the generally accepted explanation for "inadequate demand" for scrap. We now try to develop a sense of what the statement means in terms of economic consequences. Figure 7-5 suggests a significant change in the socially optimum recycling rate—from R to R^*—when a correction is made through regulation, subsidization, or taxation, for previously unaccounted-for social costs. Suppose, however, that the conventional wisdom about scrap demand is correct. What if scrap demand is indeed constrained by scrap output quality? If this is the case, demand is constrained by the inability of both scrap processing and/or steel-making technologies to remove the undesirable tramp contaminants. This situation is diagrammed in figure 7-6. This more sophisticated representation of the supply and demand relationship has profound implications for policy. As can be clearly seen from the figure, reforms directed at improving scrap demand, whether in the form of a direct

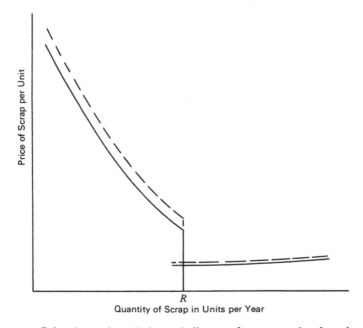

FIGURE 7-6. A supply and demand diagram for one grade of steel scrap—incorporating the hypothesis that demand is currently constrained by the presence of impurities in scrap. Dashed lines indicate comparable supply and demand functions when social costs are internalized by steel and steel scrap industries (but not by auto industry). R designates recycling rate under current laws.

subsidy or in the form of effluent charges or regulations on residuals discharges (for the steel and steel scrap industries), may well have almost no effect on demand for ferrous scrap.

Information is not yet available to allow determination of the demand curve.[29] However, from the considerations discussed in this study, it is clear that the break point in the demand curve is inexorably linked with the amount of contamination in the steel scrap being sold. It is obvious that the vertical segment of this demand curve will occur at a low value on the abscissa for a highly contaminated scrap, such as No. 2 Bundles, at an intermediate value on the abscissa for a moderately contaminated scrap, such as Shredded, and a high value on the abscissa for a totally uncontaminated scrap, such as No. 1 (construction steel is an example).

Figures 7-5 and 7-6 consider the cases of demand unaffected by impurities and demand constrained by impurities as well as the effects of internalizing social costs for steel companies and steel scrap processors. A third supply-and-demand diagram arises when the possibility is considered of internalizing the social costs imposed by the admixture of nonferrous metals in the manufacture of products made primarily of steel, such as the automobile. If the social costs of this "steel using" process are considered, the abscissa of the totally inelastic portion of the Pareto optimal demand curve is shifted to the right when the social costs are internalized, as is shown in figure 7-7. The explanation for this shift is that, were the social costs of the admixture of impurities to be internalized, either less impurities would be admixed, or they would be admixed in such a way as to ensure their profitable removal by dismantlers. Given the engineering characteristics of current scrap processing technology, a decrease in impurity level of the processed scrap would almost certainly be the result.

This brief discussion of the supply and demand for scrap indicates what should be the major concerns in studying the ferrous recycling problem. They are (a) contamination in the scrap products, (b) the potentials of reducing the contamination through scrap processing technology (at a cost), and (c) the extent to which the scrap, steel, and steel-consuming industries are internalizing all production costs.

THE QUALITY PROBLEM

Previous discussion has emphasized the desirability of minimizing impurities in scrap, given products and processes of steelmaking. Consider copper as a surrogate variable for contamination generally. Five separate scrap purification processes may be identified from our discus-

---

[29] *Ibid.*

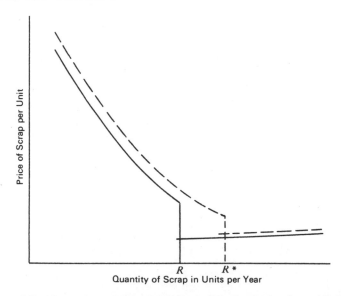

FIGURE 7-7. A supply and demand diagram for one grade of auto-derived steel scrap incorporating the hypothesis that demand is currently constrained by the presence of impurities in scrap. Dashed lines indicate comparable supply and demand functions when all social costs, including those imposed in auto production by the admixture of nonferrous metals, are internalized. R designates recycling rate under current laws, R* designates Pareto optimal recycling rate.

sion. These are hand dismantling followed by baling or shearing, hand dismantling followed by shredding, hand dismantling followed by processing in a shredder of improved design (as discussed in chapter 4), hand dismantling followed by cryogenic shredding, and hand dismantling followed by melting under high vacuum. Product characteristics resulting from these five processes are summarized in figure 7-8 and table 7-2. These summaries indicate a functional relationship between

TABLE 7-2. Scrap Product Characteristics as Related to Processes[a]

Process (including hand dismantling as usually practiced)	Estimated total cost[b] of production in dollars per gross ton	Percent heterogeneous copper removed	Percent copper in final product
Baling or shearing	18	50	0.50
Shredding	28	70	0.22
Improved shredding	30[c]	80–85	0.12
Cryogenic shredding	35[c]	90–95	0.08
Melting under high vacuum	68–80[c]	100	0.05

[a] Assumed hulk cost $10; assumed deregistered auto cost to dismantler $10; assumed hulk transportation cost $5.

[b] Cost exclusive of transportation of processed scrap and of profits.

[c] Very rough estimate—no data available.

copper concentration in the steel scrap product and the cost of the product. Points on the function which are not defined by specific processes can be defined as linear combinations of available processes.

A similar function can be defined for the dismantling process alone. To do this, it is merely necessary to vary parametrically the constraint on copper concentration in the hulk from 0.50 weight percent (which it will be if the dismantler acts in his economic self-interest—with no constraint on copper concentration) down to about 0.05 weight percent.

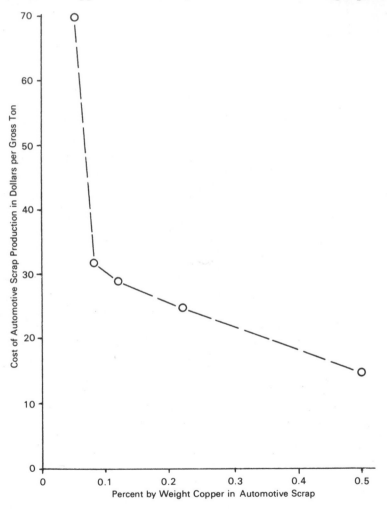

FIGURE 7-8. Estimated costs (exclusive of profit) of steel scrap produced from automobiles as a function of the amount of copper in the resulting scrap (cost estimations and assumptions same as those of chapter 6). All plants assumed to be sufficiently large so that further reductions in costs by increasing scale are negligible.

TABLE 7-3. Results of Parametric Analysis Run on Constraint on
Dismantled Hulks

Upper limit on copper concentration in metal in hulk (weight percent)	Pounds copper in auto hulk exit dismantling	Gross profit to dismantler (dollars)	Additional cost incurred by constraint (dollars per car)[a]
0.50	10.94	11.45[a, b]	—
0.48	10.60	11.44	0.01
0.46	10.15	11.43	0.02
0.44	9.70	11.42	0.03
0.42	9.25	11.41	0.04
0.40	8.80	11.40	0.05
0.38	8.35	11.39	0.06
0.36	7.90	11.37	0.08
0.34	7.46	11.34	0.10
0.32	7.02	11.32	0.10
0.30	6.58	11.29	0.15
0.28	6.14	11.27	0.18
0.26	5.70	11.24	0.20
0.24	5.26	11.22	0.23
0.22	4.82	11.19	0.26
0.20	4.38	11.16	0.28
0.18	3.94	11.11	0.34
0.16	3.50	10.98	0.46
0.14	3.05	10.77	0.68
0.12	2.62	10.55	0.89
0.10	2.18	10.34	1.11
0.08	1.74	10.11	1.34

[a] That is, forgone profit.
[b] It is assumed that the deregistered auto is purchased by the dismantler for $10, and that the hulk is sold by the dismantler for $10. The profit arises from the sale of the parts as secondary material. The radiator alone weighs about 14 pounds, which at $0.28 per pound is $3.90 (minus trivial labor costs). The engine weighs about 450 pounds, and cast iron sells for about $0.01 per pound, representing a profit of nearly $4.50 (again, labor costs are small). The battery is worth $0.65, and most secondary copper, such as wire, is worth about $0.37 per pound. Thus not much dismantling is required to attain an $11 profit.

The results are shown in table 7-3. The marginal cost of removal (that is, the cost over that incurred in producing a hulk containing 0.50 weight percent copper) of *all* the heterogeneous copper- (and yellow brass-) bearing parts is surprisingly low, about $1.34 in all.

This result is of interest for two reasons. First, analyses of No. 2 Bundles published in the literature[30] show a large variance in the concentration of copper present. As a specific example of this phenomenon, one dealer was interviewed who was producing sheared scrap containing 0.18 percent copper. The general result (a large variance) would be expected if the variation in cost with respect to final copper concentration is low. And this is indeed the case, as demonstrated by the data in

[30] See W. L. Swager, *The Measurement and Improvement of Scrap Quality* (Battelle Memorial Institute, 1960), appendix A, p. 22.

table 7-3. The marginal cost of removing those parts which would be required to reduce copper contamination to that level is only about $0.35.

Second, the data in table 7-3 suggest that hand dismantling is the least costly way to remove copper to very low levels. The marginal cost of decreasing copper concentrations from 0.50 to 0.22 weight percent (which shredders produce) is only about $0.26 per automobile if a hulk weighs about one gross ton. Even if a $3.50 per hulk charge is added to this for the cost of baling or shearing, and a $5 per hulk charge is added for transportation, the total cost of the processed scrap would be only about $19 per gross ton. The purity of the product would seem to be nearly the equivalent of the shredded material. This is not quite the whole story because the dismantled and baled product will contain a significant amount of nonmetallic (mostly organic) material. Nevertheless, the data suggest strongly that the lowest cost route to low copper at present is hand dismantling.[31]

The strength of this conclusion is only slightly diminished if the more realistic problem of constraining the five nonferrous metals of greatest interest to the steelmaker is considered. When the sum of the five nonferrous elements is parametrically constrained, the results are as shown in table 7-4. For the sake of comparison, a shredder produces ferrous scrap containing about 0.46 weight percent of the five metals. The cost of hand dismantling to the same purity level as shredded scrap is less than $2. Again, about $3.50 per car must be added to the cost for baling or shearing, and $5 for transportation so that the total cost of the product would be about $20.50 ($10 for hulk + $2 for extra dismantling + $5 for transportation + $2.50 for processing) as compared with $28 for the shredder.

The obvious question is: if hand dismantling is a very low-cost method of reducing nonferrous metallic impurities, then why is it not employed? The answer probably lies in the difficulty of enforcing quality standards in scrap purchased from dismantlers. If steel companies integrated backward into scrap production, they might be able to maintain the quality control aspects of the situation sufficiently well to guarantee any reasonable contamination level in their No. 2 Bundles. But instead, the cars are dismantled by small independent groups of individuals, dispersed over a wide geographic area. A bundle cannot be analyzed except at large cost to a steel company. Therefore the steel industry cannot depend on the quality—and will not pay a premium for ostensibly (but not identifiably) higher quality scrap. There is no economic incentive

---

[31] This conclusion is only seemingly at odds with Adams' conclusions for the same problem. He concluded that hand dismantling was the less effective technique because he included the cost of incinerating the automobile, whereas we do not. Product prices were nearly, though not quite, the same. See appendix A to this chapter.

TABLE 7-4. Results of Parametric Analysis Run on Constraint on the Sum of
Copper + Chromium + Molybdenum + Nickel + Tin—Exit
Automobile Dismantling Step

Upper limit on concentration of of nonferrous metals in hulk (weight percent)	Pounds nonferrous metal in auto hulk exit dismantling step					Profit (dollars per car)	Additional cost (dollars per car)[b]
	Cu	Cr	Mo[a]	Ni	Sn[a]		
1.06	10.94	8.78	0.65	1.34	1.30	11.45	0.00
1.00	9.98	8.78	0.65	1.34	1.30	11.42	0.02
0.94	8.59	8.78	0.65	1.34	1.30	11.39	0.05
0.88	7.23	8.78	0.65	1.34	1.30	11.33	0.12
0.82	5.90	8.78	0.65	1.34	1.30	11.25	0.19
0.76	4.56	8.78	0.65	1.34	1.30	11.18	0.27
0.70	4.12	7.89	0.65	1.33	1.30	11.09	0.36
0.64	3.87	6.80	0.65	1.31	1.30	10.97	0.47
0.58	3.57	5.77	0.64	1.29	1.30	10.54	0.91
0.52	3.54	4.48	0.64	1.27	1.30	10.06	1.38
0.46	3.51	3.20	0.64	1.25	1.30	9.58	1.87
0.40	3.49	1.93	0.64	1.22	1.30	9.00	2.45
0.34	2.69	1.43	0.64	1.22	1.30	8.39	3.06

[a] These values are deceptive. Dismantling does not remove the Mo since it is mostly present in dissolved form in the steel. Dismantling probably removes tin, however (shredding probably does so too), since the tin is mostly in the solder in the electrical equipment and the radiator and heater core. However, the *exact* location of a particular amount of tin is not known, hence the model erroneously indicates that it is not being removed. This defect in the model is a consequence of the corresponding defect in the data on the location of tramp metals in the auto.
[b] That is, forgone profit over optimum dismantling.

for a scrap dealer to remove the contaminants, since what he is paid has no relation to quality. While, as has already been noted, in some instances dealers do supply scrap of extraordinary quality, the more general rule is a wide variation in quality.[32]

The conclusion that hand dismantling is the lowest cost method of removing copper applies to the hand dismantling–shredding process as well as to the hand dismantling–baling process. For, once a few of the items containing the largest amounts of copper have been removed from the automobile, it is likely that a shredder will remove a relatively constant fraction of the remaining heterogeneous copper. Thus, if a car were initially dismantled to the 0.24 weight percent copper level, after shredding it would probably contain about 0.12 weight percent copper,[33] and the additional cost incurred over the cost of ordinary shredded scrap would be only $1 to $2.

As is the case with hand dismantling and baling, the problem with

[32] Swager, *Measurement and Improvement of Scrap*.
[33] The dismantling model constructed herein (see chapter 5) utilizes figures for the metallic components of each automotive part, the weight of each part, and the time required for its removal and dismantling, obtained from the study of automobile dismantling by Dean and Sterner (U.S. Department of the Interior, Bureau of Mines, *Construction and Testing of a Junk Auto Incinerator*, by C. J.

hand dismantling and shredding is one of implementation. The shredder operator has no assurance that dismantling to the 0.24 weight percent copper level has indeed occurred, and hence there is no way for him to give the dismantler an economic incentive for reducing the copper level.

Combinations of dismantling followed by some further processing are not likely to occur if left to the marketplace. What is needed is a process that does not need constant analytical surveillance to ensure scrap product quality. To an extent, of course, this is what a shredder offers. A steel company can, with only minor exceptions, buy shredded product from any shredder processor and be assured of a quality product. An "improved shredder" as discussed previously, could probably build up, with relative ease, a reputation for a reliable high quality product, as could processes involving cryogenic shredding and melting under high vacuum. In turn, this would presumably induce higher prices for these scrap grades. If not, then the higher quality would have to be judged as having zero marginal economic value. That this may be the case is clearly implied by the fact that shredded scrap prices are the same as No. 1 Heavy Melting scrap prices, even though No. 1 Heavy Melting has much lower impurity levels.

Dismantling and Labor Costs

The ferrous scrap industry is a labor-intensive industry, and the most labor-intensive subsection of the industry is hand dismantling. Thus it is only reasonable to expect that profits from dismantling may vary appreciably with labor costs. To evaluate the effect of labor costs on profits, eight runs were made with the dismantling model (chapter 5).

Chindgren, K. C. Dean, and J. W. Sterner, Bureau of Mines Solid Waste Research Program, Technical Progress Report 21, 1970). This study gave composite figures for ten dismantled cars of several makes ranging from 1954 models to 1965 models. The cars varied considerably in price and design and included sedans, hardtops, convertibles, and station wagons. No computer runs were made in which the values used were varied within a plausible range (that there are ranges can be readily observed from the work of Ralph J. Stone, *Copper Control in Vehicular Scrap*. Report to the U.S. Department of the Interior, Bureau of Mines, Contract No. 14-09-0070-382, pp. 66–69, 81–83.) It is clear that the model could be used for an in-depth exploration of automotive design and its effect on nonferrous contamination levels in the hulk, given sufficient funds and time. This should be done.

Suppose that, through essentially chance design modifications, the contamination level of shredded scrap were to drop from 0.22 weight percent copper to 0.15 percent copper by weight over a period of years. This would imply a change from about 0.48 percent copper by weight in the hulk to about 0.3 percent copper by weight. (This is about the largest change we could imagine arising from purely chance design modifications.) How would scrap steel buyers, the steel companies and the foundries, respond to this gradual downward change? It would seem that they might respond in a conservative fashion, that is, buy no more scrap than they ever did because of the threat of random product contamination.

All of these runs were made at prevailing labor costs and secondary material prices (see appendix A). In four of these runs the sum of the impurities[34] in the dismantled hulk was constrained to be greater than some parameterized percentage, for example 1.44 percent, 1.40 percent, and so on down to about 1.06 percent. In the other four runs, the sum of the impurities in the dismantled auto hulk was constrained to be less than some parameterized percentage, for example, 1.06 percent, 1.02 percent, to about 0.40 percent. When no constraint such as these was employed, the car was dismantled to the 1.06 weight percent impurity level. Thus the parameterized runs were necessary to determine the variation in costs with the degree of dismantling.

Each set of two runs was for a given labor cost, e.g., $6 per hour. This labor cost, however, was not taken as a simple labor cost, but included, as legitimate charges to the firm, the factors commonly added to wages.[35] Thus, for example, for a basic unskilled labor wage of $3.75 per hour, 33 percent is added to account for fringe benefits (hospitalization, vacations, etc.), raising the effective labor costs to $5 per hour. Then 20 percent is added for supervision, raising the effective labor cost to $6 per hour. This is approximately the current effective labor rate for the Philadelphia area.

Runs were made, for the two sets of parameterized nonferrous metal concentration constraints, at each of four *effective* labor rates—$4, $5, $6, and $7 per hour. The results are shown in table 7-5 and in figure 7-9.[36] The calculations dramatically illustrate the effect of labor costs in the dismantling sector of the automobile scrapping process (all other factor prices were held constant—including the sale prices of all the

---

[34] Copper, nickel, chrome, tin, and molybdenum.

[35] M. S. Peters and K. D. Timmerhaus, *Plant Design and Economics for Chemical Engineers* (McGraw-Hill, 1971).

[36] The values calculated for $4 per hour labor costs may initially appear to be in error, but in fact they are correct. The $17.06 profit per car results from the fact that when contamination levels are constrained to be greater than or equal to some value, say 1.20 weight percent, the calculations indicate that the greatest profit can be earned by dismantling the car entirely. While this initially appears to be anomalous, it fulfills the constraint imposed. To see this, let

x_1 represent the total weight of the hulk in pounds
x_2 represent the total weight of the tramp metal in pounds. Then the constraint is:

$$x_2 \geq 0.0120 \, x_1 \quad \text{or} \quad x_2 - 0.0120 \, x_1 \geq 0.0$$

This constraint is obviously satisfied by $(x_1, x_2) = (0.0, 0.0)$; that is, complete dismantling. Thus dismantling the car entirely (so that the weight of the remaining hulk is zero and the weight of tramp elements is zero) satisfies the constraint.

When this constraint is removed, the calculations indicate that slightly higher profits can be obtained by not dismantling the car entirely. That is, at 1.06 weight percent, the constraints changed from "the sum of the impurities must be greater than or equal to 1.08 weight percent" to "the sum of the impurities must be less than or equal to 1.06 weight percent."

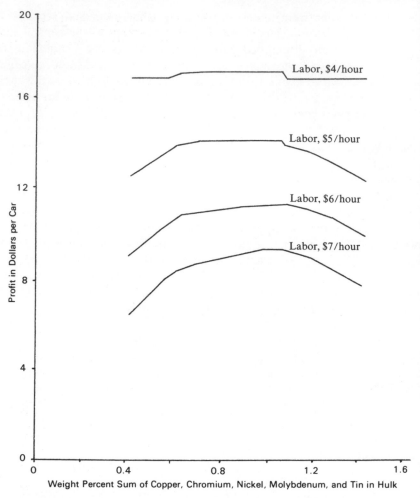

FIGURE 7-9. Dismantling profits as a function of contamination level, with labor costs as a parameter.

products derived). The runs made raised two major points. First, as labor rates increase,[37] as they have in the recent past, from $4 to $7

[37] Of course, the force of the argument hinges on the constancy of other prices and costs, such as the price of the recovered materials. Only a lengthy historical analysis of price levels would provide a completely satisfactory answer to the extent of the decline in dismantler profits with increasing labor costs. However, consider the years 1968–1972. Appendix A, which considers product prices, compares prices for 1968 compiled by Dean and Sterner (*Construction and Testing*) with those for 1972 (compiled for this study) and finds that secondary materials prices have actually dropped, on the average, in the intervening years. Thus, it can be said with a good deal of assurance that, since labor costs have almost certainly risen $1 per hour since 1968, dismantler profits have fallen about $3 per auto in the 1968–1972 period, or about 20 percent.

TABLE 7-5. Dismantling Profits as a Function of Contamination Level with Labor Cost (Including Supervision and Overhead) as a Parameter[a]

Weight percent of sum of copper, chromium, molybdenum, tin, and nickel	Gross profit to dismantler in dollars per car			
	Labor $4/hr.	Labor $5/hr.	Labor $6/hr.	Labor $7/hr.
1.44	17.06	12.46	10.02	7.73
1.40	17.06	12.68	10.24	7.95
1.36	17.06	12.89	10.45	8.18
1.32	17.06	13.11	10.67	8.40
1.28	17.06	13.32	10.89	8.63
1.24	17.06	13.50	11.02	8.85
1.20	17.06	13.67	11.14	9.06
1.16	17.06	13.84	11.26	9.18
1.12	17.06	13.96	11.37	9.27
1.08	17.06	14.06	11.43	9.37
1.06	17.38	14.27	11.44	9.45
1.04	—	—	—	—
1.02	17.38	14.27	—	9.45
1.00	—	—	11.43	—
0.98	17.38	14.27	—	9.43
0.96	—	—	—	—
0.94	17.38	14.27	11.39	9.35
0.92	—	—	—	—
0.90	17.38	14.27	—	9.27
0.88	—	—	11.33	—
0.86	17.38	14.27	—	9.17
0.84	—	—	—	—
0.82	17.38	14.27	11.25	9.07
0.80	—	—	—	—
0.78	17.38	14.27	—	8.97
0.76	—	—	11.18	—
0.74	17.38	14.26	—	8.84
0.72	—	—	—	—
0.70	17.35	14.22	11.09	8.72
0.68	—	—	—	—
0.66	17.32	14.18	—	8.59
0.64	—	—	10.97	—
0.62	17.25	14.03	—	8.45
0.60	—	—	—	—
0.58	17.11	13.76	10.54	8.16
0.56	—	—	—	—
0.54	17.07	13.49	—	7.77
0.52	—	—	10.06	—
0.50	17.07	13.23	—	7.39
0.48	—	—	—	—
0.46	17.07	12.96	9.58	7.01
0.44	—	—	—	—
0.42	17.07	12.69	—	6.57
0.40	—	—	9.00	—

[a] Assumption is that dismantler buys the deregistered auto for $10, and sells the hulk for $10. The profit is from the parts salvaged and sold.

per hour, maximum profits decrease from approximately $17.50 to $14.25 to $11.50 to $9.50 (assuming constant prices for all products and all other costs). These downward shifts in profit for relatively small increases in labor costs (really amounting to only about $0.625 per hour for the labor—excluding the 33 percent increase for benefits and the 20 percent for supervision) probably say a good deal about the incentives for a dismantler (or an auto parts dealer) to carry out the final stages of dismantling. The incentive for dismantling decreases year after year, unless there are secondary material price rises which compensate for increasing labor costs. (There were significant increases in secondary materials prices in late 1972 and early 1973.)

Suppose, for example, that wage rates are now $3.75 per hour (that is, $6 per hour labor costs) and are increasing at a rate of 5 percent per year. In less than 3 years, labor costs will have gone up to $7 per hour, and, assuming all other factor costs constant, the dismantling profits will fall about $2 per car, or about 20 percent.

Table 7-5 and figure 7-9 illustrate yet another point: that the variations in profit with contamination level (a) are relatively small for a fairly wide range of concentrations and (b) increase with increasing labor rates.[38] The former point has been discussed previously, noting that it explains the wide variation in contamination of No. 2 Bundles. As for the increase in variation of costs with respect to contamination level, these increase with increasing labor costs. This increase, coupled with long-term trends in materials prices, suggests that the day will soon arrive when dismantling will almost always consist of removing only the radiator, heater core, and battery. Other than that, only those parts which the scrap processor insists on being removed will be removed.

CALCULATION OF REMOVAL OF HETEROGENEOUS NONFERROUS METAL BY SHREDDERS

With data on the amount of tramp elements remaining in a hulk after dismantling (calculated from the dismantling model), the approximate amount of the tramp elements dissolved in the steel body, and the composition of shredded scrap, the percent removal of heterogeneous nonferrous and nonmagnetic metals by a typical shredder can be calculated (table 7-6). It is concluded that shredders remove about 60 percent of all the tramp metal that they could.

---

[38] The condition is that the selling price of a dismantled hulk is independent of quality level.

TABLE 7-6.   Calculation of Percent Removal of Heterogeneous Nonferrous
and Nonmagnetic Metals in a Shredder

Element	Wt. % tramp element exit dismantling step	Wt. % dissolved in metal	Wt. % hetero- geneous form	Wt. % in typical shredded product	Calc. percentage of removal of heterogeneous metal
Copper	0.49	0.05	0.44	0.22	50
Chromium	0.39	0.06	0.33	0.16	67
Molybdenum	0.03	0.03[a]	0.00	0.02[a]	—
Nickel	0.06	0.06	0.00	0.10	—
Tin	0.05	0.01	0.04	0.021	50
Total	1.02	0.21	0.79	0.462	~60

[a] The discrepancy between these two figures must be caused by measurement errors, which are recognized as a serious problem.

REGULATIONS ON DISCHARGE OF RESIDUALS

In the dismantling process, a large number of residuals are produced which have an unknown environmental significance. They include oil, gasoline, ethylene glycol, methanol, and sulfuric acid, some or all of which are probably poured on the ground during dismantling. While all of these are included in the dismantling model, in the present state of environmental studies, external costs could not be assigned to them. Solid residuals are also produced during dismantling, and a cost of $6 per net ton has been assigned for their transportation and disposal. This $6 per net ton is considerably higher than the numbers that were given in interviews. Nonetheless, this figure was used because it seemed to be a fair value.[39]

In the aggregated scrap processing model, provisions are made for charging for or regulating the production of sulfur dioxide, carbon monoxide, and nitrogen oxides (all produced during either open burning or incineration). Provisions are also made for charging for solid waste disposal at the rate of $6 per net ton, again at least twice the cost reported by any operator visited. On this basis, the cost per car for solid waste disposal is about $1.23, and the charge per gross ton of processed scrap is about $1.60.

In Philadelphia, air pollution particulate production is regulated by statutes[40] which relate the allowable discharge rate to the rate at which

[39] It has been argued by Calvin Lieberman of ISIS (personal interview with Calvin Lieberman, Ace Steel Baling, Inc., Toledo, at company offices, December 23, 1971 and May 12, 1972) and others that solid waste should be charged for on the basis of volume instead of weight. Provision is made in the model for charging on either basis.

[40] City of Philadelphia, Air Management Regulation V of the Air Pollution Control Board (1971). See p. 16.

material is being processed. The relationship is nonlinear. If 1,000 pounds per hour of material are being processed, the allowable discharge rate is 2.80 pounds particulates per hour; if 2,000 pounds per hour, it is 4.14; if 3,000 pounds per hour, it is 5.10. If 60,000 or more pounds per hour of material are being processed, the maximum allowable discharge rate is 40 pounds of particulates per hour. This amounts to 83,200 pounds particulates per year, assuming a 2,080-hour year. This figure is utilized in the model for the shredding plant, and the reduced cost for that row is 0.0046 dollars per pound of dust removed, which indicates a cost per gross ton of processed scrap produced of about 7 cents (assuming 15 pounds of dust produced per automobile processed).[41]

As of late 1973, some shredder manufacturers are passing the exhaust gases from the cyclone separator into a venturi scrubber. While a cyclone separator may separate 90–95 percent by weight of particulate matter, a venturi scrubber will separate yet another 90–95 percent of particulate matter, for a total particulate removal level of 99–99.5 percent by weight. Total cost per automobile (about 0.75 gross tons of shredded scrap) is on the order of $0.15 to $0.20.

It may be concluded that, while even stringent pollution control regulations (or effluent charges) would not add significantly to the cost of producing scrap, they can take up a surprisingly large proportion of the profit derived, since their investment cost may be as much as 10–15 percent of the total cost of the installation.

---

[41] Process engineering equipment is usually conservatively designed, and the cyclone separator design was done accordingly. It was nominally designed for 2.5 tons, or 5,000 pounds of entering dust per hour. The actual amount of entering dust is about 900 pounds per hour (90 autos per hour times 10 pounds dust/auto). If there are 20 pounds dust/auto, this would be about 1,800 pounds per hour.

This may seem highly conservative (a possible 150 to 200 percent overdesign) but (a) process engineering equipment is always overdesigned (normally by 25–100 percent, depending on equipment type, the cost of design conservatism, and so forth) and (b) the 10–20 pounds dust per auto figure never seemed established as well as an engineer would like. Thus, I overdesigned considerably (knowing that in this case the cost of conservative overdesign was relatively small), thinking it better to err on the high side in terms of dust removal cost.

The removal cost of $0.0046/pound for dust, or about ½ cent per pound, seems reasonable in view of the extreme simplicity of the equipment and its low manpower requirement.

Appendix A
Materials and Labor Prices

1. Labor. Going labor rates in the Philadelphia area for scrap yard workers are about $3.00–4.50 per hour or $3.75 on an average. Assuming a 33 percent figure for benefits, and assuming an overhead and administration factor of 25 percent payroll, there is a total labor cost for dismantling of $5 at a minimum (no overhead and administration) and a figure of as high as $6.25 per hour if overhead and administration are included. (Figures are based on conversations held with scrap dealers and Peters and Timmerhaus.[42]) The actual value used in this study in the auto dismantling model is $6. An equivalent value is used for the process analysis model.

2. Shredded scrap. Based on the comments of the shredder operators interviewed, shredded scrap sells for the same amount per gross ton as No. 1 Heavy Melting. Data from *Iron Age* for the price of No. 1 for the 6 years 1966 through 1971 indicate an average yearly price for No. 1 of $31.32. The average monthly price for the first 9 months of 1972 was $35.05. The figure used in this study is $31.50. The range which should be studied, based on the yearly average data, is $25 to $40. Figure 7-10 shows the history of the price of No. 1 Heavy Melting and No. 2 Bundles in graph form.

It is unfortunate that the price of shredded scrap is not listed in *Iron Age*. Analysts have been forced to use the price of No. 1 Heavy Melting as a surrogate variable for the price of shredded scrap, with no objective assurance that this approach was valid. Since January 1970, however, the Bureau of Mines monthly Mineral Industry Surveys have listed the exports of both No. 1 Heavy Melting scrap and shredded scrap, as well as the declared dollar value of the shipments before loading (onto ships). Thus it is possible to compare the dockside value of No. 1 Heavy Melting and shredded scrap. We have done this for monthly data from January 1970 to June 1973. The mean dollar value per net ton for that period was $39.03 per net ton for No. 1 Heavy Melting and $39.10 per net ton for shredded scrap. The respective standard deviations were $6.43 per net ton and $6.99 per net ton. A test of the

[42] See Peters and Timmerhaus, *Plant Design and Economics for Chemical Engineers.*

hypothesis that the values of the two types of scrap at dockside are different indicated that the hypothesis must be rejected. That is, the use of No. 1 Heavy Melting prices in lieu of shredded scrap prices is correct procedure.

3. No. 2 Bundles. Data from *Iron Age* show that the average price of No. 2 Bundles for the 6 years preceding 1972 was $20.37. The monthly average price for the first 9 months of 1972 was $23.21. The two cases of No. 2 Bundle price and No. 1 Heavy Melting price cannot be neatly separated. First, the severe fluctuations in the price of each (see figures 7-10, 7-11) result in the necessity to choose some sort of

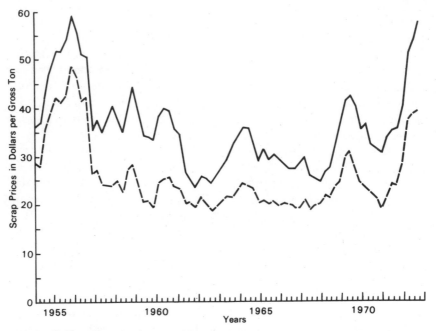

FIGURE 7-10. History of scrap prices in dollars per gross ton. Solid line, No. 1 Heavy Melting; dotted line, No. 2 Bundles.

meaningful average price for each type of scrap. Second, a review of historical trends of the data indicates that the difference between the price of No. 1 Heavy Melting and No. 2 Bundles is, though a random variable,[43] best approximated as simply a constant. In the usual nomen-

[43] The statistics for the monthly average differences are, for 213 points (monthly averages since January 1955), a mean of 9.98, a standard deviation of 3.06, a lower quartile of 7.99, an upper quartile of 12.20, a minimum of 4.00, and a maximum of 20.40. The 20.40 point appears to be a "sport," the next highest values being two at 16.00, one at 15.00, two at 15.75, and so on. A histogram run on the data gives no further insight. The distribution does not resemble any of the standard types.

clature, if c_k represents cost of scrap k, Δc represents $c_1 - c_2$, and ϵ represents a random variable with a mean of zero and variance σ

$$\Delta c = k + \epsilon$$

The mean value of Δc is \$9.98. A good sense of the situation can be gained from figure 7-12, which is a graph of the relationship between Δc and time.

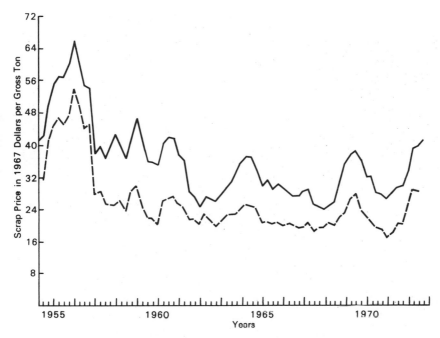

FIGURE 7-11. History of scrap prices in constant (1967) dollars. Solid line, No. 1 Heavy Melting, 1967 dollars; dotted line, No. 2 Bundles, 1967 dollars.

This cursory analysis of ferrous scrap metal commodity market prices illustrates the need to relate the price of shredded scrap to that of No. 2 Bundles. If, as indicated in section 2 immediately above, a (starting) price of \$31.50 for shredded scrap is chosen, there is a strong argument for setting the price of No. 2 Bundles at \$31.50 minus \$9.98, or about \$21.50. Moreover, when parametrically varying the price of one, it is clearly prudent to vary the price of the other simultaneously.

4. No. 2 Sheared Auto Stock is sold under prices listed in *Iron Age* for No. 2 Heavy Melting, which averaged \$7 per gross ton below No. 1 Heavy Melting for 1971 and 1972 (calculated by one data point for

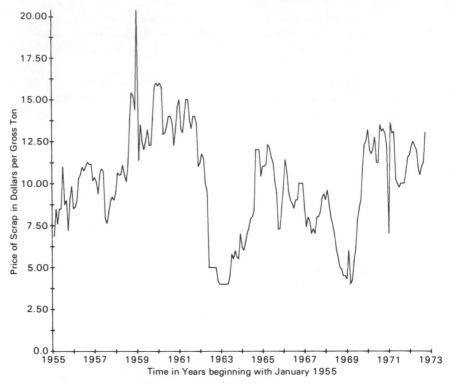

FIGURE 7-12.   History of scrap prices since 1955. Line designates difference in price between No. 1 Heavy Melting and No. 2 Bundles.

each month). The value chosen for this study is therefore, $24.50.[44] Again, this price should be varied along with the others when ferrous prices are parametrically varied in the model.

5.   Burned sheared scrap premium over sheared auto scrap is $0.00 in the Philadelphia area.[45] Therefore, the price assumed is $24.50 per ton.

6.   Burned No. 2 Bundles. The going price for these in the Phila-delphia area averages about $6 less than the price of No. 1 Heavy Melt-ing. Therefore, the assumed price is $25.

7.   Cast Iron. Averaging one data point for each month for the years

---

[44] In the dismantling model, it was assumed that the price of sheared or bundled —that is, prepared—No. 2 steel (this would be the product of a completely dis-mantled and processed auto) is $24.50 per gross ton minus an assumed necessary $4 per gross ton required preparation cost (shearing or baling) minus an assumed $5 per gross ton for shipment. That is, $24.50 − $5.00 − $4.00 = $15.50 per gross ton.

[45] This information is from purchasing agents (for steel companies in the Philadelphia area) who chose to remain anonymous.

1971 and 1972 indicates that the difference in price between No. 1 Heavy Melting and "Breakable Cast" is about $2.90 per ton (but with a large variance—*Iron Age* prices). Therefore, the assumed price for the model is $28.50 per gross ton.

8. Nonferrous metals. The prices of nonferrous metals also vary significantly over time. Rather than unquestioningly accepting the most quoted data, that from Dean and Sterner[46] (used by Adams in his study[47]), a short review was made of prices from early 1971 to early 1972 for each of the prices listed in *Iron Age* magazine. Those prices were then averaged. Then five dealers who had been particularly cooperative in previous interviews were contacted by telephone and asked what they considered the average price to be. They were not told of the averages already calculated until they gave their own estimates. Finally, all these figures, along with those of Dean and Sterner, were tabulated in tables 7-7 and 7-8 to allow ready comparison. In those cases in which the survey of five dealers agreed with the average of the *Iron Age* quotations, the average was chosen for use in the study. In the other cases, the estimate was based on the comments of the dealers.

In the case of pricing zinc die castings, considerable aid in setting realistic prices was given by W. Simon, who provided some idea of prices in the zinc die casting industry in lieu of information from *Iron Age*.[48]

9. Motor blocks. Telephone interviews were made with three scrap dealers and one broker in the Philadelphia area to determine the price for undisassembled engines (that is, an engine as pulled from the car). The results are shown in the table below.

| | Price in dollars/pound | |
| | At seller's | At buyer's |
Interview	location	location
Scrap dealer No. 1	—	0.0095
Scrap dealer No. 2	0.0075	0.0121
Scrap dealer No. 3	0.0090	—
Broker	—	0.0138

A typical shipping price would be about 0.00125 dollar per pound. This suggests a price to large-volume sellers of 0.01 dollar per pound or

[46] See U.S. Department of the Interior, Bureau of Mines, *Dismantling a Typical Junk Automobile to Produce Quality Scrap*, Bureau of Mines Report of Investigations 7350, 1969.

[47] Adams, "An Economic Analysis of the Junk Automobile Problem."

[48] Walter Simon, Delaware Valley Smelting Corp., Tullytown, Pa., personal communication, October 23, 1972.

TABLE 7-7. Prices of Nonferrous Metals in Dollars/Pound

Metal	Data effective												Avg.
	1/4/71	2/1	3/1	3/29	5/3	5/31	6/28	8/30	10/4	11/1	11/29	1/3/72	
Copper:													
Radiator stock	0.26	0.24	0.265	0.315	0.305	0.29	0.295	0.29	0.2775	0.2725	0.25	0.255	0.276
No. 2 hvy. and wire	0.37	0.355	0.385	0.425	0.425	0.365	0.385	0.375	0.355	0.355	0.32	0.35	0.372
Yellow brass solids	0.24	0.235	0.255	0.295	0.285	0.25	0.25	0.25	0.24	0.235	0.21	0.22	0.247
Zinc, die castings	—	—	—	—	—	—	—	—	—	—	—	—	—
Aluminum, cast, etc.	0.1275	0.1325	0.1325	—	0.1325	0.1325	0.130	0.225	0.1225	0.1175	0.1175	0.1125	0.126
Lead:													
Battery (prices per battery)	0.725	0.675	0.675	0.675	0.675	0.675	0.675	0.675	0.675	0.675	0.525	0.525	0.654
Battery cable clamps[a]	0.0425	0.0375	0.0375	0.0375	0.0375	0.0375	0.0375	0.0425	0.0425	0.0525	0.0575	0.0575	0.04025

[a] In this case it seems clear that the price quoted from *Iron Age* magazine is not related to the price in the "marketplace" in which we are interested.

TABLE 7-8.   Prices in Dollars/Pound Established by Dealers or Buyers

Metal	Dealers					U. S. Bureau of Mines—1968[a]	Values chosen for this study
	A	B	C	D	E		
pper:							
Radiator stock	0.29	0.31	—	0.29	0.31	0.3275	0.276
No. 2 heavy and wire	0.30	0.38	—	0.39	0.41	0.396	0.372
Yellow brass solids	0.29	0.28	—	0.27	0.275	0.31	0.247
nc, die castings	0.12	—	0.065	0.05	0.09	0.0625	0.06
uminum, cast, etc.	0.12	0.12	—	0.11	0.11	0.124	0.126
ad:							
Battery (price per battery)	—	—	—	0.55	0.65	1.40	0.654
Battery cable clamps	—	—	—	0.11	0.11	0.11	0.11

[a] U.S. Department of the Interior, Bureau of Mines, *Dismantling a Typical Junk Automobile to oduce Quality Scrap.* Bureau of Mines Report of Investigations 7350 (Washington, D.C.: Government Printing Office, 1969).

more, and about 0.009 dollar per pound to small sellers. The latter price is used in the model.

10. Copper-bearing stock. Items such as motors and generators are often sold as "copper-bearing stock." The current price for this material in the Philadelphia area is about 1¼ cents per pound of material (of which of course only a relatively small fraction is copper).

11. Auto hulks. Prices offered for auto hulks seemed to cover a wide range for the dealers with whom the issue was discussed. For example, $18 per net ton *delivered*, $15 per net ton *delivered*, and $10–20 per net ton *delivered*. The figure used in the calculations that were performed was $10 per hulk (a hulk weighing almost exactly a gross ton, depending on the assumptions made about the disposition of glass and other sundry items) *at the dismantler's site.*

8

Perspective

RECYCLING FERROUS MATERIAL

This study has presented a detailed engineering/economic study of that segment of a regional steel scrap industry that uses obsolete automobiles as raw material. The elements of this "system" include: the availability of deregistered autos, hand dismantling to remove salable parts, scrap contamination, methods of scrap processing and their costs, prices of scrap products, transportation of both raw scrap and processed scrap, profits, and residuals generation and management. This chapter attempts to view the scrap problem in perspective.

Basically the recycling problem should be viewed in the context of alternative sources of raw materials to meet the demand of society for goods and services at any time. Demand includes the particular characteristics or specifications of the goods desired, both intermediate and final. These specifications in turn affect the combinations of raw materials and production processes which can be used to meet the specifications.

The relative proportions of residuals (that is, scrap) versus virgin raw materials (that is, iron ore) used is a function of their relative prices. Relative prices are affected by at least three major variables: (a) the technology of raw materials processing, both for steel scrap and iron ore; (b) the costs of managing the residuals generated in the processing and use of raw materials; and (c) the various tax assessment and transportation pricing policies affecting the alternative raw materials. Thus, the degree to which ferrous material is recycled is a function of these major variables. This study was limited to a study of the scrap alternative raw material and focused on the first two variables cited above.

Research Results

The research reported here furnishes new and explicit information on obsolete automobiles as a source of ferrous material. This information has important implications for various policies which propose increases in the degree of recycling.

First, while it is shown that the short-term elasticity of supply of automobile steel scrap, at market equilibrium, in geographical regions near large cities has been fairly high in the past, it is probably increasing with time, because of the development and gradual adoption of improved technology in collecting and transporting obsolete automobiles. This research suggests that short-term supply elasticities could be as high as 5–10. This result strongly suggests increased and more sophisticated attention to the demand side of the problem.

Second, it is shown that there is substantial potential for the development of scrap processes capable of producing higher quality scrap at only slight additional processing cost. Realization of this potential will occur only if there is a sufficient price differential for higher quality scrap. Evidence obtained during the research indicated that at the present time such a differential is essentially nonexistent within a given nominal grade class, apparently because of the inability to analyze scrap. In the case of shredded scrap, the typical product may now be so pure as to result in a zero marginal value of more processing.

Third, the research indicates quantitatively the extent to which nonferrous materials in steel products affect the costs of processing the products to obtain ferrous raw material. This finding emphasizes the important effect of final demand on recycling.

Fourth, this study strongly suggests that the residuals discharge associated with automobile scrap processing can be reduced at relatively low cost as compared with the residuals discharge associated with iron (from blast furnace) production. Thus, an increase in demand for scrap might be expected if all raw material producers had to pay the total social costs associated with their residuals generation.

Fifth, although this research has not concentrated on the transportation problem, the models developed have incorporated transportation costs to the steel mill or foundry, thus making it possible to study in detail the effects of this key variable on the flow of scrap material. Moreover, the research has demonstrated the important effect the costs of transportation from the source of the obsolete scrap to the scrap processor have on supply elasticity—an aspect of the transportation problem that has received insufficient attention in the past.

The Use of Scrap in Perspective

Referring back to figure 1-1, it can be seen that this study has covered in depth only one of the many links in the recycling chain—the ferrous scrap industry which uses deregistered automobiles as a raw material. What is clear is that the entire system is highly complex and that there are some major unanswered questions. Most of these questions relate to the demand for scrap, which is the other factor—in addition to supply—which affects the extent of recycling.

The demand for steel scrap as a raw material is of course a function of the price of scrap. But price in turn is affected by various technological (and economic) factors associated with use of scrap and other ferrous raw materials and the characteristics of the steel and steel products produced. These factors include:[1]

1. The mix of furnace types used in the steel industry, since the open hearth, the electric furnace, and the BOF processes have different capacities for using scrap
2. The product mix of steel production; if a larger fraction of the steel produced had less severe constraints on nonferrous content, the quality constraints on use of steel scrap would be less restrictive
3. The price of prereduced ore, which serves as a constraint on the maximum level scrap prices can reach, since they are substitutable goods, even in an electric furnace
4. The design of motor vehicles, and other goods, in terms of the proportion of nonferrous materials included and their forms, that is, separable or inextricably mixed

Among the unanswered questions, and hence logical topics for research, are the following:

1. What proportion of the total number of obsolete automobiles is currently processed to obtain ferrous material? How does this vary by region?

2. What is the current disposition of steel scrap produced from obsolete automobiles? What proportions comprise inputs into various steel production process types and steel output combinations? For example, is most of this steel scrap input to electric furnaces for the production of lower quality steel products?

---

[1] See W. J. Vaughan, "A Linear Programming Approach to Residuals Management in the Iron and Steel Industry," Ph.D. dissertation to be submitted to the Department of Economics, Georgetown University, Washington, D.C., 1974; see also C. S. Russell and W. J. Vaughan, " A Linear Programming Model of Residuals Management for Integrated Iron and Steel Production," to appear in *Journal of Economics and Environmental Management*, vol. 1, no. 1.

3. How does the design of automobiles explicitly affect the costs of processing obsolete automobiles and the quality of scrap produced? What are the effects of annual model changes and multiple styles of a given model on processing costs? To what extent does the increased complexity of automobiles—engine size and design, automatic transmission, power equipment, air conditioning, electric windows, etc.—affect processing costs and scrap quality?

4. What are the specific technological limits on the quantities of steel scrap of different qualities which can be used to produce different steel products by different processes, that is, steel furnace types?

5. For the same steel production process–product output combination, how does the contribution of steel scrap to overall residuals generation and residuals management costs compare with that of virgin ore?

In addition to these basic technological–economic questions, there are some important economic policies which affect the relative use of the two alternative raw materials, and hence the extent of recycling. Steel scrap and iron ore as alternative raw materials apparently receive differential economic treatment, as indicated in the following remarks by Representative Martha W. Griffiths:[2]

FEDERAL INCOME TAX DISCRIMINATION AGAINST RECYCLED SOLID WASTE MATERIALS

The hearings before the Subcommittee on Fiscal Policy made it clear beyond doubt, however, that recycling will never be able to play its proper role unless and until the Federal Government acts to remove or modify all of the existing economic impediments to recycling which it has unfortunately fostered over the years.

By far the most important of these impediments is Federal income tax discrimination against recycled materials. Presently, the income tax laws, which provide, first, capital gains treatment on income derived from the increase in value of timber and second, the percentage depletion allowance applicable to the extractive industries, favor the utilization and depletion of virgin natural resources over the utilization of recycled materials.

In the case of metals, percentage depletion allowed under the Federal tax laws places virgin metal ores in a more advantageous competitive position than recycled metals. Percentage depletion for iron and copper is 15 percent of gross income, while for most other metals the depletion allowance is 22 percent. In addition, there is a special tax provision similar to the timber (sic) capital gains treatment which applies to the disposal of domestic iron

[2] See U.S. Congress, House, Representative Martha W. Griffiths speaking for the House bill for recycling incentives, H.R. 15770, 92 Cong., 2 sess., June 30, 1971, *Congressional Record*, E 6629-2230.

ore. Because of these special tax provisions, mining industries have a much lower effective tax rate than manufacturing industries. The 1969 Treasury Department Tax Studies show that the mining industries, excluding petroleum, have an effective tax rate of only 24.3 percent of net income as opposed to 43.3 percent of other manufacturing companies. A company which uses recycled metals will fall into the higher bracket manufacturing category. Again, therefore, integrated metal manufacturers and smelters are rewarded by the Federal tax laws for continuing to deplete our dwindling virgin ores while the recycler is penalized for taking actions which alleviate the solid waste problem and conserve virgin resources that are becoming increasingly vital to our national security and welfare.

These economic policy issues are addressed in detail by Page.[3]

Several policy conclusions follow from all of the above. First, for a given final demand, that is, the mix and specifications of final products, and given technology of steel production, various incentives by federal and state governments to increase use of obsolete steel scrap—subsidies of one type or another to scrap processors and/or users—may have little or no impact on the extent of recycling. The technological constraints implied by given production process–product mix may impose a relatively low upper limit on demand.

Second, the removal of the existing preferential economic treatment of iron ore, compared to scrap, would permit the market to establish the most efficient level of recycling (assuming all externalities were internalized).

Third, it is not clear how the extent of scrap recycling would be affected by the enforcement of strict constraints on discharges of gaseous and liquid residuals to the environment. Scrap processors appear already to have reduced their residuals discharges, at low cost, to relatively low levels. This does not appear to be as easily done for some iron ore producing and processing operations. In addition, steel producers will be differentially affected by residuals discharge controls, especially because there is a wide variation in the extent to which individual steel plants have already responded to effluent controls. Further, foundries—major users of steel scrap—produce large quantities of particulate matter and are facing major additional costs to meet air quality standards. Determining how these various interacting forces will affect recycling requires further and more comprehensive analysis, including an analysis of the extent to which use of steel scrap of higher quality would reduce residuals generation and residuals management costs at steel mills.

[3] Talbot R. Page, "Economics of Recycling," in *Resource Conservation, Resource Recovery, and Solid Waste Disposal,* Committee print 93–12, Senate Committee on Public Works, 93 Cong., 1 sess., (1973), Resources for the Future, Inc., 1973.

In sum, what is needed is an analysis of the total system for producing steel, with: (a) various degrees of recycling; (b) various combinations of steel production processes; (c) various degrees of scrap processing; (d) various designs of products using steel, and thus various mixes of steel outputs; and (e) costs of required residuals management at all points in the system. Such an analysis would allow the explicit determination of the effects of alternative economic policies and technological constraints on the use of scrap and the extent of recycling.

Index

THE JOHNS HOPKINS UNIVERSITY PRESS

This book was composed in Times Roman text and display type by Maryland Linotype Composition Co., Inc. It was printed on Warren's 60-lb. Sebago, regular finish, and bound in Holliston Roxite, by The Maple Press Company.

Library of Congress Cataloging in Publication Data

Sawyer, James W
  Automotive scrap recycling: processes, prices, and
prospects.
  Includes bibliographical references.
  1. Automobile wrecking and used parts industry—
United States.   I. Resources for the Future.
II. Title.
HD9710.U52S28   338.4'7'6285   74-3101
ISBN 0-8018-1620-3